DIY

Signature Perfume Creating
Subtitle   **Why Natural Is Best**.

Author Robyn Ji Smith

Compendiums to this book
- Alluring Study Of Aromatherapy By Robyn Ji Smith
- Learn Perfume Creating - Subtitle Organic & Synthetic Series 6 Edition 4 By Robyn Ji Smith

Before chemistry, was a science, before chemistry and science -there was alchemy, both are experimental. This is your journey, experimenting with aromas that will uplift your mood and excite others. Enjoy.

Choose your mood and design your natural scents to suit. This book covers the principals of natural perfume designs, plus alcohol based and the new laws that are causing perfumers around the world massive headaches. Included are the websites that control the new laws.
Making perfume at home is very easy as long as you understand the blending tables, mixing rules and contra-indications of essential oils. All of which you will find right here in these informative pages.

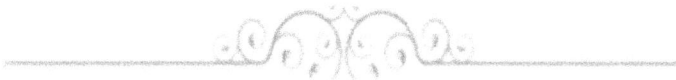

Why Natural Is Best

DIY Signature Perfume Creating

Sub tile: Why Natural Is Best

by

Author Robyn Ji Smith

Printed by Robyn Ji Smith
At KDP Amazon

Publisher **Beauty School Books Of Beauty Pathways Academy Book 1 of Series 6 Edition 4**
http://www.beautyschoolbooks.com.au

ISBN 9780987506542

Copyright

DIY Signature Perfume Creating

Index

Why Natural Is Best

Why Natural Is Best

Why Natural Is Best

The most expensive Perfume in the world to date is Shumukh at $125,500,000

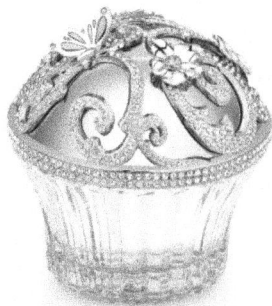

But my favourite bottle after Chanel No. 5 is Cheery Garden by the House of Sillage at $1650

By Robyn Ji Smith   page. 8

DIY Signature Perfume Creating

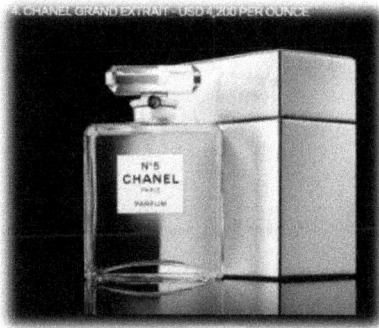

My favourite shaped bottle is Chanel No. 5. I also love the story on how Coco Chanel hired a Chemist and he created Chanel No. 5 by accident. He added too much absolute.

However, the aromas are now mostly synthetic as there are new laws to prevent being used in perfumes. So perfumes will never again smell like they once did.

Will the big guys still get to cheat on our vulnerable natures and our health? Oh yes, because governments tax perfumers highly and there is too much to lose.

I am passionate about doing the right thing and people either love or dislike that about me. Now my children are in their 50s my daughter told me to lighten up or not come to her luncheons. Well that was a good vent Bub, I said. LOL *Note, she still asks me every week. Kids…. Mmmm.*

With that said, you can rest assured I am not going to willingly lead you astray just to sell a book. Loads of things are changing in the perfume industry and its all tight lip from perfumers but I will do the research and pass it on to you.

This video on YouTube gives just a filter of the new laws.

https://www.marketwatch.com/story/the-4200-bottle-of-perfume-2013-05-10

Everything In Life Is A *Journey*

I pray this book is the beginning of a marvelous journey for you.

Let us begin with the important issues - Blending for healing and safety

Blending Measurements For Organic Perfumes

First do not get tablespoons and teaspoons confused.
There are 85-115 eyedrops of essential oil to 1 teaspoon of essential oils. This is equal to 5ml or $1/6^{th}$ of an ounce.
Drops can differ with oils, eyedropper and Dripolators.
There are many ways to calculate and scales often measure incorrectly.
For aromatherapy calculations my students liked this method and I found it works well when you need to measure butter, powders and oils to ascertain the safe amount of essential oil to use. we do it like this:

Blending -Calculations Made Easy – 1%to 5%

How calculate 1%, 2%, 3%, 4% and 5%

Calculate the mass weight have a look at the table below on tablespoons to milliliters and milliliters to grams. The abbreviation in recipes or on medication bottle is Milliliters- abbreviated either ml or mils

Essential oils are added by drops, therefore to calculate the drops of a 1% blend we need to calculate our carrier.
100 ml of let us say olive oil is

1oo x 25= 2500 drops
1% of 2500 drops is done on the calculator like this
2500x1% = 25
This means 1% of essential oils in a 100ml size bottle of carrier oil is 25 drops.
And two (2%) is 50 drops of Essential Oil in 100Ml of carrier oil. One percent is for the face and two percent is the strength of essential oils in a carrier oil for the body.
But what if you have a recipe that has 6 **table**-spoons of arrowroot powder
10 table-spoons of shea butter and 1% of essential oils. You can work it out with **table 3** below. But I want you to try and learn your conversions.

Calculate like THIS:-

6 Tablespoons of arrowroot is equivalent to approximately 89 milliliters or 89 grams in weight. So, if we always try to remember that essential oils are worth 25 drops as 1% of 100 ml of carrier or 50 drops is 2%
So 89 ml or 89 grams multiplied by 25 = 2225
2225x1% = 22.25 drops so we would use 22 or 23 drop of essential oil with the 6 tablespoons of arrowroot

Let us now add 6 tablespoons of Arrowroot and 10 tablespoons of Shea butter.

This is 16 tablespoons of product.
In table 3 below we see 1 tablespoon is equivalent to 15 milliliters or 15 grams we multiply the 16 tablespoons by 15 grams = 248 grams
Multiply 248 grams by 25 =6000
6000x1%= 60 so we now know that 16 tablespoons of product can have 60 drops of essential oil added at 1% dilution
Or if we want it for be a body butter and tell people is suitable for the body only.
We would do the sum like this
6000x2% =120 drops of essential oils

Why Natural Is Best

For perfumes soap you may add 3 to 5 percent of essential oil compound. Let us say your soap ingredients in total comes to 750 grams after adding the liquids and solid ingredients together and have called them grams.

1. You multiply the grams by 25 (750x25=18750)
2. Put 18750 in your calculator press the times button (x) button and the 3, or 4 or 5 button and
3. the percentage button (%)
4. then the equals button (=)

Now you have - how many drops of essential oil you need. For 3% you need 562 drops. But to stand and count all those drops you are bound to get it wrong. So, you would use teaspoons. Which is about 5 and a half teaspoons. See table 2.
Less is always best when safety is your main priority.

The calculator online conversions are not always correct Eye droppers and dripolators depending on the thickness of the oil can weigh differently. Also, unless you have a very good quality science type of scales it is almost impossible to weigh small drops of essential oils correctly.
When the recipe calls for you to measure the ingredients in ounces use an ounce to milliliter conversion table. See table 4

This is the table (table 1) I was given in college and I was very satisfied with it because I was only dealing with essential oils and blending them with base oils and I trusted my teacher.

Table 1

Carrier	Essential Oil For Body 2%	Carrier	Essential Oil For Face 1%
100 ml	50 drops	100 ml	25 drops
50 ml	25 drops	50 ml	12 to 13 drops
25 ml	12 to 13 drops	25 ml	10 drops
20 ml	10 drops	20 ml	5 drops
10 ml	5 drops	10 ml	2 drops
5 ml	2 drops	5 ml	1 drop

It is very important to work out which way you are going to measure your signature/perfume compound as it is the signature compound that you will be adding to your base to complete your perfume.

This table is for **teaspoon** size measures. So, if you use eyedropper there is 100 tiny eyedrops in 1 teaspoon. One hundred eyedrops (100 eyedrops) is double the safety amount of essential oils you can add to 100ml of carrier oil, for a massage oil. So, you definitely do not want to be adding essential oils via a teaspoon into your products.

Table 2

Table A Essential Oil Equivalents in Measures -tsp= Teaspoons			
100 drops Of Eos	1 tsp	5ml	1/6 ounce
200 drops	2 tsp	10ml	1/3 ounce
300 drops	3 tsp	15ml	1/2 ounce
400 drops	4 tsp	20ml	2/3 ounce
500 drops	5 tsp	25ml	5/6 ounce
600 drops	6 tsp	30ml	1 ounce

Tablespoons to Millilitres to Grams Approximate Measures,

This table is important when you begin to make a recipe with mixed ingredients. Such as butter, powders, base oils, water and alcohols.

Table 3

Approximate Measures, Tablespoons to Millilitres to Grams

Tablespoons ➡ = Millilitres		Millilitres oil ➡ To Grams	
1	14.79	15	15
2	29.57	30	30 (28.35g) =1oz
3	44.36	45	45
4	59.15	60	60 = 2 oz
5	73.93	74	74
6	88.72	89	89 = 3oz
7	103.51	103	103
8	118.29	118	118
9	133.08	133	133
10	147.87	147	147
11	162.65	162	162
12	177.44	178	178
13	192.22	192	192
14	207.02	207	207
15	221.88	220	220

Warning teaspoons in your kitchen vary in size. From 60 to about 110 drops. If you are going to use spoons as your measure buy the baker measure. If you use milliliters and eyedropper blending tables you will not need to worry. Do not get confused this is not the safety drop to use in a blend. The above teaspoon chart is about how many eyedrops of essential oils there would be in a teaspoon. Never use a recipe that states how many teaspoons of essential oil to use. See Blending *Tables*

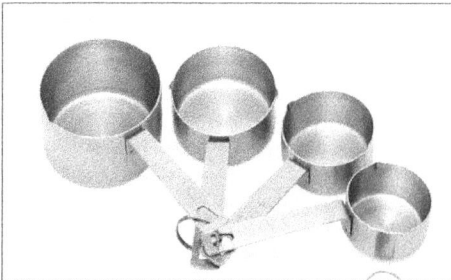

DIY Signature Perfume Creating

When using powders as your carrier you will probably find recipes that have tablespoons or grams. A recipe might tell you to add a carrier oil or a powder such as arrowroot by tablespoons. I pray when you finish reading this book you will know how to calculate percentages safely. You will also explore making perfume compound and know the safety rules.

Once you start exploring how to blend essential oil aromas - to make a compound or signature aroma to add to other products such as dusting powders, body butter and so on you will **not** need other peoples' recipes.

Table 4

Fluid Ounces	Millilitres
1/4	7
1/2	15
1	30
2	55
3	85
4	115
5	140
6	170
7	200
8	225
9	255
10	285
11	315
12	340

I will make a video on this soon and upload to my channel

Here are some already made on my channel

https://www.youtube.com/user/beautyschoolbooks/videos

Be Marvelously Alive.   **15** | P a g e

Blending For Body

Recommended blending for the body, is a 2 to 2.5% dilution of essential oil to the carrier oil. This means one drop of essential oil to every two (2) mills of carrier oil. Or about 50 drops to 100ml.
OR
Just follow the blending table.
As we use essential oils by the drop and most recipes tell us to add 1% to 5% depending on the product you are making.

Blending For The Face
When blending for the face the dilution is 1.25% this is exactly half of the body quantity of essential oils/drops. But for easy mixing and safety we use 1%

Blending For Pregnancy And Baby
In Pregnancy the dilution is 1/2% (half) to 1% never stronger and only after the 3rd month unless a practitioner and a doctor OK it. Babies only after the 6th month as their liver isn't yet formed and only with a Doctors or Practitioners guidance.

Making Blends For A Diffuser

There is no need to add a base oil for a blend to go into a diffuser. It is best to only have 1 to 3 oils in a diffuser.

Kaolin and Talc
Adding your signature perfume to Talc/Arrowroot or Kaolin clay (powder) is a wonderful way to add layers of perfume to your body.
Be sure to add some uncooked rice to the jar to prevent the talc or clay from clogging or balling. To a 200g jar of clay I add about 100 drops of my signature perfume Compound.
Read more in the recipes test section on this subject.

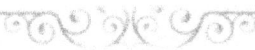

Blending Considerations

These same rules in measure pertain to blending natural perfumes be they cream based (emollients) or Carrier oil-based perfumes.

With alcohol-based perfume this blending table does not really apply. But the laws are changing and I will be guiding you through a safer method of mixing with an alcohol-based perfume.

Alcohol is known as a fixative in perfume making. When deciding on which essential oils to use in mixing the Signature compound, known professionally as the **perfume compound** for the less natural alcohol-based perfumes you do not need to worry as much about the fixative type essential oils, nor the quantity of the Signature/perfume compound.

Blending for home use is different to blending products to sell. You may be happy to have a preservative free product but when you start selling to strangers all the rules change. I have added information in this book about ratios. Tag the important pages, so you can go straight to the information when required.

Contamination considerations

Now we are embarking on recipes and blending safely, I feel the need to explain. With any product that requires you or a customer to dip into
the jar - with fingers or a spoon, equals possible contamination. How can you guarantee that the customer or you or a family member will always use a clean soon?
With any product that requires you or a customer to dip into with hands or a spoon equals contamination problem.

When reading the recipes consider these facts.

Why Natural Is Best

Dipping your fingers into a jar can contaminate it with bacteria. Moisturizer textures can be so luscious and tempting! —but it's not really a good idea to stick your fingers into a jar. Doing so will contaminate the formula with bacteria that is invisible to the naked eye. Can we educate our customers to use a clean spoon every time they dip-in. Probably not.

We have options.
1. Do not make retail products that people dip into.
2. Add preservatives to the product.
3. You can make body butter more liquid by adding more carrier oil. This affords the benefit of putting them into a bottle with a pump top, in place of a jar.

Blending Calculations
Water Based Recipes

Water in any product needs to be considered the enemy. Water used in the formulation of cosmetics is not your everyday, regular tap water. It must be 'ultra-pure'—that is, free from microbes, toxins, and other pollutants. For this reason, your label may refer to it as distilled water, purified water or just aqua.

When a recipe calls for water, you **need to use distilled water**

When adding essential oils to a water-based product - you must first render the essential oils miscible, before adding to the water.

At proper concentration, ethanol/95% Alcohol "marries" essential oils and water together, so they become one homogeneous substance that can no longer be separated into two distinct substances. There can be no separation or 'divorce', they're forced to stay together for good! Consider high proof "Everclear" as your alcohol of choice until you learn more.

Alcohol to essential oil ratio

The ratio is 1 in 4. 1 drop of essential oil to 4 drops of alcohol. This is the safest way to blend essential oils when adding them to a water-based recipe. If the recipe fails to tell you this you now know what to do.

Body Blending Oil Or Perfume Blending

Lest say you have made your perfume compound in your test bottle. It will be transferred to dark glass. but this photo is so you can see what is happening.

You want to make a natural perfume, in 50ml bottle. You almost fill the bottle with not 50ml but about 49ml of carrier oil. You then take your pipette and take 25 drops of the perfume compound and add to the 50ml of carrier oil.

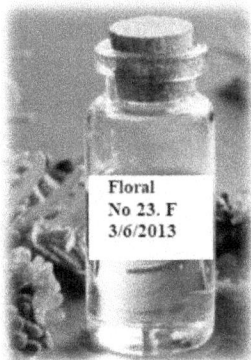

Floral
No 23. F
3/6/2013

Blending Table
Body-Blending Table
Carrier - Essential Oil for the body can be as low as 2% is recommended as a healing method.
Carrier - Essential Oil
100 ml - 50 drops
50 ml - 25 drops
25 ml - 12 to 13 drops
20 ml - 10 drops
10 ml - 5 drops
5 ml - 2 drops

Face Blending Table.
Carrier - Essential Oil for the face 1%
100 ml - 25 drops
50 ml - 12 drops not twelve and a half drops as less is best.
25 ml - 6 drops

Be Marvelously Alive.　　　**19** | P a g e

Why Natural Is Best

   20 ml - 5 drops
   10 ml - 2 drops
   5 ml - 1 drop

   Pregnancy Blending Table.
   Carrier - Essential Oil for Pregnancy 1/2% (Half a percent).
   After 3rd month
20 ml Of Carrier Oil - maximum is 2 drops or less
30 ml - maximum is 3 drops or less
50 ml - maximum is 5 drops or less

   The above blending tables are the way you mix essential oils with a base oil such as olive oil, almond, grapeseed, or jojoba.

   However, in perfume blending you might use 1 or 2 drops of essential oil or perfume compound to each milileter of carrier/base oil

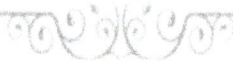

Blending Table Charts

The Alluring Study Of Aromatherapy For Healers and Perfumers

BLENDING TABLE CHART

The face and neck skin is thinner and more sensitive than the rest of the body. Therefore, the mixtures should be at half strength.

Body Blending Table - for the body 2%   Face Blending Table 1%

Carrier Oil	Essential Oil For Body	Carrier Oil	Essential Oil For Face
100 ml	50 drops	100 ml	25 drops
50 ml	25 drops	50 ml	12 to 13 drops
25 ml	12 to 13 drops	25 ml	10 drops
20 ml	10 drops	20 ml	5 drops
10 ml	5 drops	10 ml	2 drops
5 ml	2 drops	5 ml	1 drop

Aged skin is half the above dose for body use face blending for face blending use half face drop quantity.

Safety – Contra-indications Info

I update my website info on a regular basis.
lhttps://skinsex.com.au/essential-oil-blending
And often on my Facebook group
https://www.facebook.com/groups/FolkloreHealings

Always patch test a new product. Place a small amount behind your ear. If and when you start a market stall offer free patch tests. It is wise to sell the product to the client and then do the patch test. Make sure you tell them if they break out and blister or the skin becomes irritated. Providing they have not opened the jar you can either swop the product or give them their money back. I, in days long gone by - would do the patch test put the product aside for them and they often did nòt return. That can cause you to worry. Did they have a reaction? They probably forgot to come back or changed their mind. Have a large copy of the contra-indication card on display. Bring their attention to it and ask the appropriate questions. If it is an all-natural product people have ailments and some oils will be a contraindication to some of them.

Contra-indications

First you need to know if any of the oils in your perfume are unsuitable for some people or yourself.

If you have a skin condition, are pregnant, have epilepsy or asthma, a heart condition, are on a course of treatment with prescribed medication, or are in any doubt about any condition you may have, you are advised to seek the advice of a doctor or certified Aromatherapist or Naturopath or another suitable practitioner before using pure essential oils.

That blurb should be in the box with the perfume you sell, along with the ingredients list. This is a set of general safety guidelines to help you use essential oils with minimal risk. And remember, risk and hazard are two different things to consider.

A few things you need to know

Be Marvelously Alive.   **21** | P a g e

Why Natural Is Best

What oils are contra-indications to health of people. I will be giving some help in this book on how to do that but these issues are out lined in **Foolproof Aromatherapy** book by Robyna Smith-Keys and one of my books called "**Alluring Study Of Aromatherapy" For Healers And Perfumers** by Robyn Ji Smith

Do not ingest essential oils unless advised to do so by a practitioner who is qualified/licensed to prescribe essential oils in this way. I myself would never ever take nor prescribe essential oils this way. My motto is they are **"nil by mouth "**

Taking essential oils orally engages many areas of risk that other methods do not. Do not take essential oils either undiluted or in water, as there is a risk of mouth/stomach irritation. This is similar - to what happens in a bath (see above) except that mucous membrane tissue is more sensitive than skin, yet our gut only sends out pain signals when erosion has progressed quite far. Essential oils are widely used in food flavorings, and GRAS status for many essential oils applies to food flavoring use, but it specifically excludes medicinal use. One or two drops of most essential oil can be safely taken in a day, once or twice a year, but more than this is not recommended. In Australia ingesting essential oils is on the banned list, by TGA and there is good reason.

Inhalation And Diffusion
It is **not** advisable to directly, nor intensively - inhale essential oils for longer than 15-20 minutes, such as with steam inhalation. However, this does not apply to ambient inhalation from essential oils vaporized into the air. If you are diffusing essential oils, it makes more sense to do this intermittently than constantly, all day long. Ideally, diffuse essential oils for 30-60 minutes on, then 30-60 minutes off.

Safety it is best not to diffuse some oil around pets and children. More on this in contraindications.

This is not only safer, but it's also more effective as both our bodies and our nervous system habituate to essential oils after this period of time. Whenever you are using or diffusing essential oils, some air exchange (fresh air) is advisable.

Asthma

Although perfumes have been known to exacerbate asthma, this has never been recorded for an essential oil, perfume. However, anecdotal accounts suggest that individuals with asthma may find that certain essential oils trigger an attack.

Naked flames

Essential oils are flammable, and should not be used in any way that involves close proximity to a naked flame or similar fire hazard. Essential oils are not explosive, and they are safe when used in a diffuser, but there is some degree of risk. Burners that are lit with a candle flame are not recommended, but fragrant candles are safe.

Children

Keep essential oils in a place where young children cannot reach them, and never let them handle essential oils bottles. Even two-year old kids have been known to unscrew caps on essential oil bottles and drink the contents. The fact that the bottle contains an orifice reducer helps a little, but young children are used to sucking liquids. This usually results in a visit to the emergency room. While the end result is rarely fatal, every year there are some very close calls.

To help prevent such accidents, all essential oils should be sold in bottles with child-proof caps. Of course, this doesn't always work, but it does make a difference.

CO_2

In perfume making it is important to note that all CO_2 oils and resins/gum are extremely concentrated by nature. They remain true in aroma to the plant material more so than other methods of extraction. They should not be evaluated in this state unless you are accustomed to the undiluted fragrance.

Why Natural Is Best

For those trying CO2 oils for the first time, we strongly recommend they be evaluated in dilution. Otherwise, the complexity of the fragrance – particularly the rare and exotic notes – become lost. It is at this stage unproven that this form of extraction has the same healing benefits as stem distillation.

Contraindication Chart - Essential Oils

Essential Oil Contraindications Chart	
Contraindications	**Avoid-Do Not Use**
Alcohol more than 3 drinks	Clary Sage
Antidote To Homeopathy Remedies:	Eucalyptus, Peppermint, White Camphor, Black Pepper
Asthma	Avoid oils high in 1,8 cineole Eucalyptus globulus and radiata (Eucalyptus globulus; Eucalyptus radiata), Helichrysum gymnocephalum, Laurel Berry. Laurel Leaf (Laurus nobilis), Niaouli ct 1,8 cineole (Melaleuca quinquenervia ct 1,8 cineole), Saro (Cinnamosma fragrans), Ravintsara (Cinnamomum camphora ct), Tea Tree.
Babies under six months	Avoid all essential oil and scented products Unless prescribed by Doctor or certified practitioner.
Bleeding Strong Menstrual Flow	Basil, Cedarwood, Fennel, Clary Sage, Myrrh, Marjoram, Sage, Peppermint, Thyme.
Blood Pressure (Hypertension per = high)	Eucalyptus, Peppermint, Rosemary, Thyme, Sage, Basil (all varieties)
Blood Pressure (Hypotension po=low)	Lavender, Clary Sage, Melissa, Marjoram, Ylang Ylang, Lemon.
Blood thinners medication, Aspirin Warfarin And Barbiturates	1,8 cineole containing oils Ravintsara, all Eucalyptuses, Rosemary camphor/ 1,8 cineole, Cardamom, Helichrysum, Laurel Leaf, Myrtle, Spike Lavender) should not be used with barbiturates. Methyl Salicylate (Birch, Wintergreen), Peppermint and Eugenol (Clove, Basil ct Eugenol) Citrus Oils
Cardiac Fibular	Peppermint and Rosemary Thyme essential oil.
Epilepsy	Basil, Eucalyptus (Globulus, Radiata & Polybractea), Fennel, Peppermint, Rosemary, Sage & Thyme.
Estrogen Patch Wearer.	Avoid Geranium, Clary sage, essential oil.
Gastric Problems:	Avoid Cinnamon, Clove and Oregano essential oil.
Inhalations, Douches, Enemas	Cajuput, Cassia, Cinnamon Bark, CO2s, Costus, Clove Bud Elecampane, Fennel, Origanum, Pine, Resins and Savory, Tea tree, Thyme.
Insomnia:	Avoid - Peppermint, Basil, Lemon Verbena essential oil and Rosemary essential oil.
Lactation: - Oils that interfere or dry up milk flow during Lactation	Clary Sage, Peppermint, Sage (blocks the milk duct)
Liver, Kidney & Urinary problems	Avoid Juniper Berry essential oil, Eucalyptus essential oil and Black Pepper essential oil.
Medications - Barbiturates A therapist must prescribe suitable oils to use safely.	When on medications avoid all Citrus essential oils, citrus fruits. & citrus juices for 4 hours after taking medication
Mucous Membrane Irritants	Thyme, Cajuput
Pregnant.	Basil, Cedarwood, Fennel, Clary Sage, Myrrh, Marjoram, Sage, Peppermint, Thyme.
Puberty In Males- May increase breast size	Lavender, Tea tree all varieties.
Sensitive Skin	Basil, Cedarwood, Cypress, Eucalyptus, Fennel, Lemon, Lemongrass, Lime, Peppermint, Pine, Tea Tree, Thyme, Ylang Ylang.
Spa Baths	Avoid Massage & all Essential oils until 30 minutes after spa
Sun and Sun Lamps- Photosensitive to some skin types.	Lemon, Lime, Orange, Verbena, Tangerine, Mandarin, Bergamot, Angelica, Lemongrass, Grapefruit.

Aromatherapist Robyn Ji Smith www.skinsex.com.au

The flip side of this chart lists the bending tables.

Why Natural Is Best

Blending For Safe Use Of Essential Oils

Carrier Oil For Body	Essential Oil For Body 2 %	Carrier Oil For Face	Essential Oil For Face 1 %
100 ml	50 drops	100 ml	25 drops
50 ml	25 drops	50 ml	12 to 13 drops
25 ml	12 to 13 drops	25 ml	10 drops
20 ml	10 drops	20 ml	5 drops
10 ml	5 drops	10 ml	2 drops
5 ml	2 drops	5 ml	1 drop

- Always Blend in Dark Glass Medicine Bottles or Jars
- Aged skin is half the above of face blending use half face drop quantity.
- Never diffuse essential oils in the same room as babies or pets

Essential Oils Added To Other Products Such As Powders And Butters
100ml or 100 grams is multiplied by 25 then by either 1 or 2 or 3 percent
100 x 25 = 2500 x 1% = 25 drops
177 ml or grams 177x25=4425 x 1 %=44.25 drops of Essential oils use 44 drops
177 ml or grams 177x25=4425 x 2 %=88.5 drops of Essential oils Half a percent
177 ml Or Grams 177 x25 =4425 x.5%=221 drops

Water And Essential Oils Do Not Blend. For a water based recipe add essential oil to 95% alcohol like Everclear® ratio is 1 in 4. One drop of essential oil must be blended with four drops of alcohol

Pregnancy Blending Table.
Carrier - Essential Oil for Pregnancy 1/2% (Half a percent).
after 3rd month
20 ml Carrier oil/body butter - maximum is 2 drops or less
30 ml Carrier oil/body butter - maximum is 3 drops or less
50 ml Carrier oil/body butter - maximum is 5 drops or less
100 ml Carrier oil/body butter - maximum is 10 drops or less

Babies over 6-12 months use half a percent as for pregnancy. We advise not to use essential oils on babies.
Use wool fat or bees wax, mixed with olive oil for nappy rash. Warm the wax and blend in the olive oil. Place in a dark glass jar. Place 1 drop only of Lavender EO on their bed under their pillow to calm them.

Post Natal Depression	SNIFF - Rose, Bergamot, Sweet Orange, or Sandalwood And Meditate.
Labour Pains	Clary Sage to start labour. Lavender to relax. Chamomile to release tension. Geranium - to expel afterbirth. Sniff Frankincense for fear. Sweet Marjoram for spasms
Morning Sickness	Sniff Peppermint. Eat raw ginger or have in a juice. Make massage oil of ginger with olive oil after 1st trimester

Produced by Aromatherapist Robyn Ji Smith
More Free Info www.skinsex.com.au

For a clear crispy copy of this very important chart, I will be placing on my website at a not-for-profit price. However, all the information with more details is in the following pages.
https://skinsex.com.au/shop/ols/products/aromatherapy-blending-essential-oils-safely-contraindications-chart
In any form of education - it is not as important, to know everything - as it is to know where to find the required information, you need quickly.

Contra-Indications –

Oils to Be Avoided -Under Some Conditions

Antidote To Homeopathy Remedies:

Eucalyptus, Peppermint, White Camphor, Black Pepper

High Blood Pressure

(Hypertension per = high) -

Do not use:- Eucalyptus (all), Peppermint, Rosemary, Thyme Sage, Basil (all varieties),

Low Blood Pressure

(Hypotension po=low) –

Do not use:- Lavender, Clary Sage, Melissa, Marjoram, Ylang Ylang, Lemon

Photosensitive to some skin TYPES: -

Lemon, Lime, Orange, Verbena, Tangerine, Mandarin, Bergamot, Angelica, Lemongrass, Grapefruit.

Photo TOXIC: -

(do not use during the day, go into sun or under a sun lamp) Bergamot, Lemon, Orange, Neroli

Epilepsy: -

Basil, Eucalyptus (Globulus, Radiata & Polybractea), Fennel, Peppermint, Rosemary, Sage & Thyme.
The oils that are convulsive or can cause epilepsy are generally made up of Phenols or Oxides which in large dosages can cause convulsions and be neuro-toxic, so correct dosages are important when blending. Phenols are the most irritant on skin and mucous membranes and they can damage liver if in massive dosages.

Pregnant.

Oils not to use in pregnancy at all:

Basil, Cedarwood, Fennel, Clary Sage, Myrrh, Marjoram, Sage, Peppermint, Thyme.

Lactation: -

Oils that interfere or dry up milk flow during lactation:- Clary Sage, Peppermint, Sage (blocks the milk duct)

Why Natural Is Best

Safe Oils For Lactation:
Lemongrass, Geranium, Fennel (1/2%-1%) **But Diluted. However, I am not happy to supply oils to women breast feeding. Offer them a carrier oil.**
To Increase Lactation:
Anise, Fennel, Lemongrass, Jasmine

However, I recommend not using essential oils while breast feeding. Use wool fat mixed with olive oil as a skin repair and nipple repairer, after a feed session and not within an hour before the next feed.

To Decrease Lactation:
Mint, Parsley, Sage.
Let us say you have added Fennel to the signature/perfume compound then you would add a warning *Avoid while pregnant and best feeding.*
A few essential oil companies say: -
"Fennel and Basil essential oil are thought to be a galactagogue and can be used to increase milk supply"
My ancestors say eat peanuts and drink water to increase milk flow. So that is what I did week one but my milk was more of an overflow. For women with not much milk, I would recommend using a milk pump after each feed. The more often the baby sucks on a breast the more milk you will produce. However, some women simply do not produce enough milk and I certainly would not recommend using essential oils of fennel nor basil while breast feeding.

OILS That Can Cause Skin Sensitization
Or irritate a sensitive skin type: - Basil, Cedarwood, Cypress, Eucalyptus, Fennel, Lemon, Lemongrass, Lime, Peppermint, Pine, Tea Tree, Thyme, Ylang Ylang..

Inhalations, Douches, Enemas
Oils " not to use" for Inhalations, Douches, Enemas:
Thyme (all varieties) Cajuput, Tea tree, Resins and CO2s

Oils that are Mucous Membrane Irritants: -
Thyme, Cajuput (comes from the Tea Tree family)

Oils that have Emmenagogic Properties: -

Emmenagogic pronounced *em·men·a·gogue*
A substance that stimulates or increases menstrual flow.
(i.e., promotes menstrual flow): - Basil, Cedarwood, Fennel,
Clary Sage, Myrrh, Marjoram, Sage, Peppermint, Thyme.
Naturally these are not safe during pregnancy. Which is a
same as peppermint is great to stop vomiting. However, they
can diffuse it.

Babies not at all

Under six months, safest for 6-month-old to 2 years: -
German Chamomile, Lavender and Mandarin (but in a 1/2%
dilution for massage) Only one drop in a bath mixed with 2 -
3 tablespoons of carrier.

Let us imagine you have a signature /compound, that you
have mixed. You love it and want to make a natural perfume.
Due to the fact most, women put perfume behind their ears
and men put it into the palm of their hand and slap it onto
their face. We would use the face blending table for adults.

Puberty In Males

A 2007 study reported that using lavender and tea tree oil
topically on males who have not reached puberty has been
linked to hormonal abnormalities that encourage breast
growth. These oils should only be administered through
aromatherapy methods or avoided. Talk to a medical
provider before using these essential oils on or around
children. Popular essential oils that should never be used on
or around infants and children:

Eucalyptus, fennel, peppermint, rosemary, verbena,
wintergreen.

Spa Bath and Bathing

Spa - Never add essential oil to a spa nor rub oils on and go
into a spa bath. The essential oils will multiply the healing
energy waves in your body by about 100 to 1000 times.

Causing a drug overdose effect in the blood stream. You can rub a massage oil on twenty minutes after your spa but no sooner as your body is pulsating much faster than normal. The vibrational energy of the spa is healing in itself you do not also need essential oils.

Bath – Never have your incandescent (Electric Run Lights) lights on when using essential oil blends - in your bath. They have odour molecules that turn toxic from the artificial lights. If night time fill your bath, light the candles, turn off the lights and soak for 20 minutes.

This information should be added to your bath oil leaflet when selling bath oils. Bath oil blends should only be 1-3 essential oils in a carrier oil. See Blending *Tables page 98*. Other helpful resources
I put info about contraindications and new oil research in my essential oils section of my website and on my Facebook group

https://skinsex.com.au/essential-oil-blending
https://www.facebook.com/groups/FolkloreHealings

Signature / Perfume Compound Blending

A compound is your signature fragrance compound/perfume
In the signature/perfume compound we need: -

1. a base note (essential oil)
2. a middle note (essential oil)
3. a top note. (essential oil)
4. Plus, a fixative - yet some essential oil automatically work as a fixative.
5. Do not use resins/gums until you have had more training.
6. It is best to buy resins that are already reduced to an oil for perfume making, unless you are making a wax or cream perfume. Resins need heat and essential oils loose aromas with heat.

Scientific perfume makers put the essential oil **base note** in first then the middle and then the top note. They do so - one drop at time for the first few drops then add extra of each note, a few drops at a time.

They shake or stir the mixture and smell as they go. They only add the fixative when they are happy with the aroma. However, a fixative, also has a fragrance it changes the aroma. They are not worried about mistakes, as they can blend again because someone is paying them to make the compound, or they have money to burn. As a beginner or home maker you might want to do it the way I did it when I started.

I have my oil "note list" printed out. In time you will know what notes are top, middle or base - without looking at your list.

I have no idea why chemists say we should put our notes into the beaker / mixing jar, base notes first, then middle, last the top notes. I can only assume base note molecules and aromas sit in the mixing jar longer than the middle and top notes. It is also important not to take too long to mix the compound

Why Natural Is Best

because the aromas are wafting out of the mixing jar and into the air.

To get the compound right and still call it natural for your sales is a very hard call. This section of the book has troubled me for weeks. How do I condense the information that has taken me many decades to learn into a small "How To Book"?

 My end thoughts are I cannot give you years of study all in one book.

I need to keep it as simple as possible - so you can all experience the joy of natural home-made perfumes. Thus, saving you a load of money and adding to the healing powers of being creative and yet still understand the main contra-indications. If people are sensitive to perfumes, they are more than likely going to be sensitive to a natural perfume as well.

There is a big difference between making a perfume for yourself and making them to sell. Begin this wonderful journey by making just a couple of products for you, and your family first and use for a trial period. Make extra and put through a stability test which we will be discussing later.

If you stick to the blending tables and learn the contra-indications of the oils you choose - you should be safe to go. Your recommendation in your leaflet should be something like this. :-

All perfumes natural or not - can cause reactions in some people. If you are sensitive to perfumes, we suggest you do as our ancestors did and wear the perfume on your petticoat, a handkerchief tucked into your bra, (brassiere}, a timber medallion or on cotton wool ball in a locket.

Next add any contra -indications for the oils you have used such as

Example

Warning this fragrance is not suitable if you are Pregnant or Lactating (breastfeeding)

This warning would go into your leaflet inside the box.
On the outside of box state: -
"Warning not suitable while pregnant".

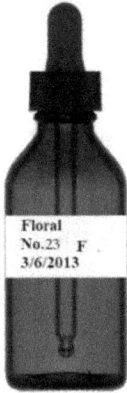

I the author Robyn have used - being pregnant as an example for you the reader/student, because in my test compound I have added oils pregnant womenfolk cannot use plus the mix of essential oil compound mix, ratio to base oil is too high.

Floral
No.23   F
3/6/2013

Don't sweat the small stuff.
Just create first for yourself.

1. First sterilize your tools and work space.
2. Make several Signature/perfume compounds
3. Document every drop you place in each test bottle.
4. Then when you have created the aroma, you love
5. Allow to sit for two days to six weeks or more so all oil aromas mellow or merge together. This is called marrying the oils.
6. Mix it with your base oil or cream. (for a more natural perfume or with alcohol for a standard unnatural perfume.
7. Hygiene- Be sure to filter your perfume and use only clean containers to store them in.
8. As soon as you have made your compound transfer into a dark narrow neck glass bottle
9. You don't want to introduce bacteria, fungi, or mould into your perfume, nor do you want to encourage their growth. Many essential oils inhibit microbial growth, so this is less of an issue with perfume. However, it can become more of a concern if you dilute the

          perfume to make cologne. Think of water as your enemy.

10. Then look up the contra- indications of the essential oils you have added to your chosen test signature/ compound. If there is an oil added that has a contraindicate, then you do not wear it on your skin. You wear it on a timber necklace or in a locket or other methods I have suggested above. And in the section heading named "**Marketing**"

After making your compound aroma transfer into a dark glass bottle for storage. If you have made 10 or more millilitres of compound you will not use all of it in one perfume. You will be adding just drops into your base. Let us say your perfume bottle is 50ml you will only use between 12 and 50 drops of compound to the 50ml of base oil. This depends on the type of perfume you are making be it, a parfum, cologne or toilette. see notes on "Perfume Percentages"

You can make an organic perfume and turn into colognes by adding alcohol. When you add water the equation changes.

Signature Perfume Test

Test Mixing

Often enough - when we read instructions, they do not make complete sense. It is important that you have read this entire book before you begin. Next, get some coloured water, bottles, talc, and some cream, and pretend you are doing what I am explaining Or, get your kit out and go through the steps, as you read.

I love to start my compounds in a clear glass jug, beaker, or bottle, because watching the perfume compound being made excites me. It is a cheap thrill but, hey, who cares every dash of happiness in life should be embraced with great delight.

DIY Signature Perfume Creating

I also start mixing when the sun catches my crystals hanging in my window. The rainbows in many places on my walls from the crystals also adds a marvelous uplift to my mood. My dog is always very excited when I wake up in the morning and loves his cuddle and a kiss. Because he is excited that I am awake - he also lifts my mood. You may think this is hogwash but your mood is very important as everything has energy.

Never store your compound in a clear glass jar or bottle always store in narrow neck dark glass.

In the morning when you wake up, you need to decide how you feel.

Be organized and at one with yourself.

Never start before you have had your cuppa, made your bed, been for an early morning walk and balanced your chakras. You're showered and dressed for success, chores are done, tick.

Be in the most marvelously alive - state of mind.

1. Organize a beautiful work space with everything you need.
2. Turn your phone onto silent.
3. Decide on which "Note Family" you are going to create. As an example, I am going to walk you through a Romantic Floral Note.
4. Have your pen and recipe book open read to write down everything you do.

Example Of A Signature Compound.

Use three to five essential oils
Put them in your test bottle or glass beaker one drop at time
and smell as you go.
I am using 4 essential oils. Aroma molecules and chemical
compounds will fight each other so less is best until you
become very familiar with your oils.

1. Start with the base notes put maybe 3 drops in your
   test beaker or bottle
2. Build with one drop of each at a time.
3. Next the middle notes
4. Next the top note
5. Shake, keep building one drop at a time, smell and
   decide.
6. Last add the essential oil you have chosen as your
   fixative. Add it one drop at a time.
7. When happy with the aroma transfer to a dark glass
   narrow neck bottle with an eyedropper.
8. Date and label the bottle
9. Two to Six week or more rest time is needed
10. Then you add it to your chosen base be that a carrier
    oil, a cream, talc or alcohol.
11. You will do this in about 3 or more test bottles, adding
    different amounts of each note. Write down what you
    are adding to each test bottle.

Here are tests I did

Base notes I had on my table were
Frankincense, Ylang Ylang, Patchouli, Vetiver

Middle Notes
Basil, Rose Geranium, Melissa

Top Notes
Bergamot, Orange, Lavender, Laurel Berry,

Lavender is classed as a top note but does the work of a base note and a fixative

My test bottles were narrow neck 50 ml Blue glass. With an eyedropper lid. For six weeks after making these signature perfume compounds, I kept in my pantry on the bottom shelve.

Signature tests 1 & 2

Test One		Test two
2 drops of Patchouli	base	3 drops Patchouli
8 drops of Laurel Berry	top	5 drops Laurel Berry
4 drops Bergamot	top	7 drops Bergamot
5 drops Lavender	Middle Fixative	3 drops lavender
1 drop Ylang Ylang		2 drops Frankincense

This is a perfume compound and must not be put onto the skin. You must now store it from a few days to weeks. Then blend it with base oil. However, I use this as a perfume in my perfume pendant on cotton wool without adding a base oil.

1. I put the base notes in each test bottle first. Adding different quantities to each test bottle. Although I have the total written here for each oil they did not go in, in this quantity, all at once.
2. Next the middle notes
3. Then the top notes
4. To tie it all together I added lavender to both tests, *I also find Frankincense and Myrrh are good fixatives.*
5. Due to frankincense being a wax you could heat slightly now and run through a coffee filter or wait for the aromas to blend *(6 weeks)* then heat gently. Sometimes the essential oil of Frankincense is

already melted into an essential oil form, with jojoba oil. This is a good way to buy it when you first begin.

However, it will often reset in the bottle and go dark. It is a tricky oil as it is actually a wax so buy from a supplier who loves their trade. You can also buy it in liquid form 3% in Jojoba base oil. When I was a beginner this is how I would buy and use it.

6. I waited six weeks for the aroma to musically blend.
7. Put through coffee filter.

All the essential oils when blended together is your compound also called an accord.

8. Then add to a base oil or a cocoa butter. base.
9. Or leave neat to use in oil diffusers/burner or in a perfume locket as smell therapy

You need to be experimental.

Natural Is A Big (?) Question

The creation of a fragrance is an excellent example of nature and science working in concert. You are the conductor. Are you going to design perfumes that do not harm people or are you making perfumes that are classed as natural but without the all-natural science added to your signature accords?

Are you going to add a few exquisite safe essential oils to a base oil known as a carrier that makes the essential oils miscible or are you going to make perfume compounds to add to other base products?

In this book I will endeavour to give you my knowledge on how to do it all ways and then you need to decide.

At this point we should look at Skin and how products in Aromatherapy enter the skin.

Skin Pathways - Perfumes

First education is the key to success.

Aromas do not last long on skin especially dry skin. All perfumes only last a few hours then you need to reapply. To understand this - you would need to study scent chemistry and that is not really necessary. Most people know they cannot smell their own perfume for long - yet friends will say you smell good several hours after the scent escapes you. A synthetic fragrance could last up to 4 hours a natural fragrance can also last that long, sometimes much longer..

Placing on the wrists and rubbing the wrists together can cause the skin to heat which produces enzymes that change the composition of the fragrance and the aroma to fly away more quickly.

A citrus compound needs a wood aroma added to hold it to the body longer on warm days. A laboratory style perfume manufacturer would add more synthetic fragrance.

When applied to the skin on a warm day causes floral and citrus perfumes to lose their crisp sent.

Perfumes and essential oils do not like temperature changes. Never place on a window ledge. Keep in a cool dark place.

They stay fresh longer at 70 degrees Fahrenheit /21.2 degrees Celsius, and do not like lights. That's why a dark glass bottle is best or keep them in their box.

Remember that perfumers have a love of money and they want yours. If your perfume is smelling off you will buy another bottle.

Steam in the bathroom causes toxins inside your perfume bottle. Never keep fragrances in the bathroom.

Why Natural Is Best

Understand that this is a skin section when seen under a microscope. This section is probably the size of a five cent coin. Skin is only 2mm-5mm thick.

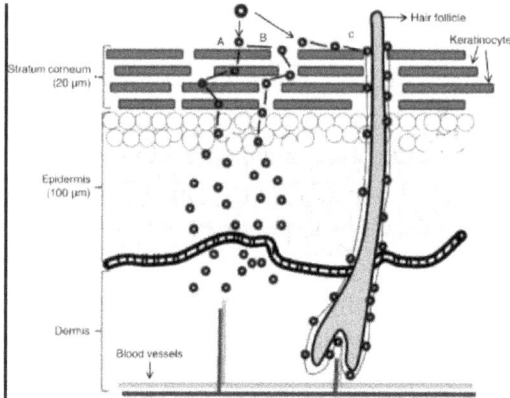

A Outter Layer
The oils head straight for the blood stream

B The oils find their way into a skin pore
C They travel down the hair follical Into the sebaceous glad then into the blood stream.

Unless you are a professional book illustrator or photographer it is hard to produce great photos for

books So look up skin photos on the web if you want to study skin in detail.

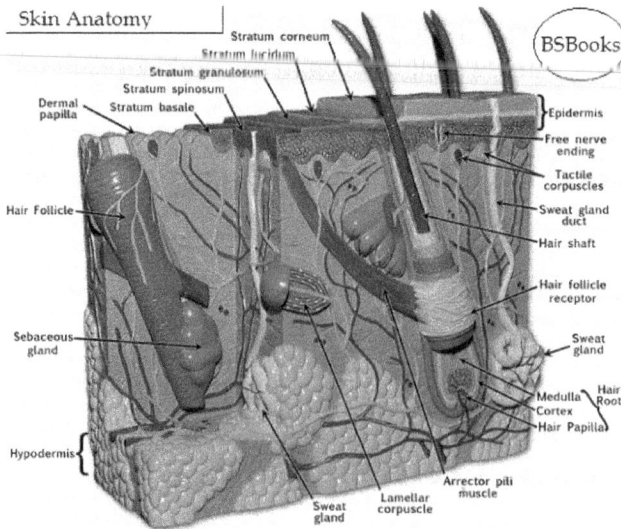

Skin Anatomy

The outermost layer of the skin is the epidermis, which is comprised of 4 to 5 layers (depending on the location in the body). stratum Corneum, stratum Lucidum (palms and soles only), stratum Granulosum, stratum Spinosum, and stratum Basale. As cells mature, they progress from the stratum basal, out toward the stratum corneum.

By the time they reach the stratum corneum, they have become anucleated and highly keratinized. The highly keratinized nature of the stratum corneum renders it a highly effective

protective barrier, especially from transepidermal water loss.

The innermost layer of the skin is called the dermis.

It consists of connective tissue, nerve endings, blood vessels, lymphatic vessels, sweat glands, sebaceous glands, and hair follicles. For the purposes of transdermal absorption, the dermis provides minimal interference. The most significant barrier of transdermal absorption is the epidermis. By the time a transdermal agent has passed through the epidermis and reached the dermis, it has now gained easy access to blood vessels for systemic circulation.

Essential Oils: The Lipid-Lovers

As their name would imply, essential oil constituents are lipophilic ("fat-loving," or fat-soluble). This suggests that essential oils mix well with oils, and poorly with water. As discussed previously, the keratinized nature of the epidermis is primarily designed to prevent desiccation/dehydration; thus, the skin is a relatively lipophilic/hydrophobic barrier. Since both essential oils and the epidermis are relatively lipophilic, essential oils and skin "mix" relatively well together; consequently, essential oils wonderfully, have a greater tendency for transdermal absorption.

Factors Influencing Transdermal Absorption of Essential Oils.

Many factors affect transdermal absorption rate and amount. Included among them are surface area of the application, location of the skin application, exposure time, use of an occlusion technique, and temperature.

Certain factors, as a general rule, have specific effects on transdermal absorption Surface Area of Application

Absorption
- Exposure Time Absorption
- Occlusion   Absorption
- Temperature Absorption

Regarding location of the skin application, areas with the thinnest epidermal layers, and areas rich in sebaceous glands, sweat glands, and hair follicles, prove to be the best areas of transdermal absorption. These locations include face, neck, scalp, and wrist.

From Skin to Blood

Research suggests that essential oil constituents are found in traceable amounts in the bloodstream following topical applications. One study conducted with lavender essential oil tested for linalool and linalyl acetate (the 2 major constituents of lavender essential oil) in the blood following a gentle abdominal massage with a 2% lavender 98% peanut oil blend. Amounts of both constituents were identified 15 minutes after the beginning of the massage, with the peak occurring around 30 minutes. The study also calculated their half-lives: 13.76 minutes for linalool and 14.30 minutes for linalyl acetate. This demonstrates that these essential oil constituents do not remain in the bloodstream for long, and are **readily metabolized** by the body thus doing their natural healing work. This is providing they have been made miscible in a base, otherwise they will sit inside the liver and stimulate the stellate cells to initiate scaring, and sit there as a harden ball.

Conclusion

Their lipophilic nature and small molecular size makes essential oil constituents great candidates for dermal absorption. In fact, their aroma molecules are able to enter the bloodstream through such topical applications in quantifiable ways.

Many factors influence transdermal absorption. By understanding the science of essential oils and the physiology of the body, we can target our therapies and maximize our aroma-therapeutic effects.

Warning

As essential oils are many thousands of times stronger than the actual herb or plant they came from, they should never ever be applied to the skin without diluting them in a carrier oil. See Blending tables pages 102 to 107

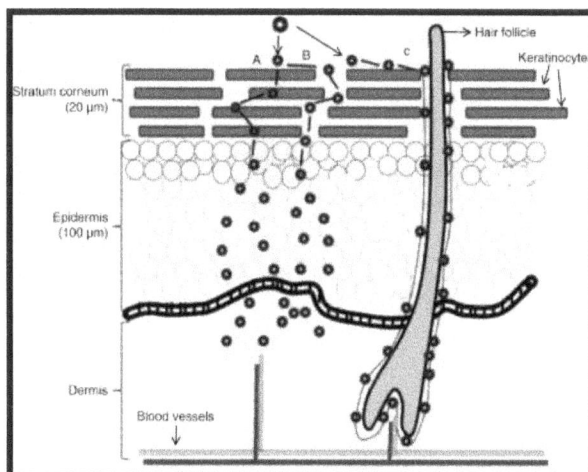

Hapten

As small molecule which, when combined with a larger carrier such as a protein, can elicit the production of antibodies which bind specifically to it (in the free or combined state). The term hapten is derived from the Greek haptein, meaning "to fasten." Haptens can become tightly fastened to a carrier molecule, most often a protein, by a covalent bond.

The hapten then reacts specifically with the antibodies generated against it to produce an immune or allergic response.

Haptens And Adverse Reactions

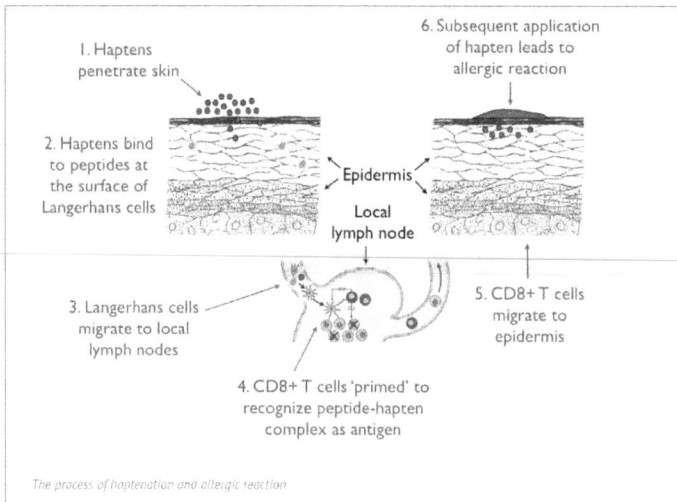

1. Haptens penetrate skin
2. Haptens bind to peptides at the surface of Langerhans cells
3. Langerhans cells migrate to local lymph nodes
4. CD8+ T cells 'primed' to recognize peptide-hapten complex as antigen
5. CD8+ T cells migrate to epidermis
6. Subsequent application of hapten leads to allergic reaction

Epidermis

Local lymph node

The process of haptenation and allergic reaction

In the aromatherapy world, the most common type of adverse reactions are skin reactions to topically applied oils. Adverse skin reactions (ASRs) are also one of the most obvious types of adverse event – when it happens you can feel it, and others can see it. ASRs are divided into four broad categories:

1. Irritation (irritant contact dermatitis)
2. Contact urticaria (immediate hypersensitivity)
3. Allergic contact dermatitis (delayed hypersensitivity)
4. Photosensitivity/phototoxicity

It has been said - that it's impossible to have an allergic reaction to essential oils, because they do not contain proteins, and only proteins can cause allergies. However, an allergen is a substance, protein or non-protein, capable of inducing allergy or specific hypersensitivity.

Mistakes DIY Perfume Makers Make.

Pure essential oils, based on their chemistry obtained via distillation will never mix with water. Their specific gravity in most cases is lighter so they will float on top.
There are many chemicals which can solubilize essential oils so they become miscible with water but only a few are on the natural side.

Glycerine
One is glycerine, a non-fermented alcohol
 which is very skin friendly, inexpensive and easy to obtain. It does not completely break down all essential oils, but does enough of a job that the essential oil is dispersed safely when adding water.

Alcohol
Alcohol, either pure ethyl alcohol (grain) or denatured alcohol which must be at least 60% while 100% (anhydrous) is optimal. Pure ethyl alcohol is strictly controlled in most countries and costs a small fortune creating a barrier for the average person to obtain.
Denatured is relatively inexpensive and not controlled, but there are few suppliers out there.

Why Natural Is Best

Once you add alcohol to a perfume it can no longer safely be called natural. Try to buy Q-Grade or perfumers' alcohol or

Sometimes we have ethyl alcohol in stock. Email Robyn
beautyschoolbooks@gmail.com

Isopropyl Alcohol
Although isopropyl will render or solubilize essential oils so they become miscible with water the aroma will be very unpleasant.

Methylated Spirits
Also known as denatured alcohol, methylated spirits is for the most part just plain alcohol (ethyl alcohol). The difference between the two alcohols is ethanol is made from grains, fruits and vegetables and methanol usually from wood stock. **But it has additives to it to stop people from drinking it and is now known as poisonous.**

You may find it in some old perfume makers books and my mum, nan, and great grandmother used it in cosmetic formulas but you can no long do that because of government regulation/interference with the product. It was regarded as a cleaning product and did not carry a big tax. New laws have made it unnatural in structure.

WARNING: Do not attempt to drink methylated spirits.

Witch Hazel
Myth - Witch Hazel is advertised to blend essential oils for skin use. This is most definitely not true. Essential oils will not be miscible when mixed with witch hazel.

Vodka
Vodka is also advertised to blend essential oils and that is untrue as well.

Aldehyde

Aldehydic Containing 13 carbon atoms with molecular formula $C_{13}H_8ClFO$, the odour profile of this aldehyde can be described as fresh, clean, soapy, citrus, waxy grapefruit peel. Its purpose is to provide watery, citrus, and floral notes to many diverse types of fragrances.

C7 – or heptanal, naturally occurring in clary sage.
C8 – octanal – which is reminiscent of oranges.
C9 – nonanal – smells of roses.
C10 – decanal – powerfully conjures up orange rind. Citral is lemons,
C11 gives a 'cleanness' to fragrance (it's naturally present in coriander leaf oil).
C12 –well, that's lilac or violets.
C13 Waxy, grapefruity.
C14…the peach-skin warmth.
Some of these aldehydes are now on the banded list.

Have a look at C8 as a study guide. click this link or just search any of the "C" numbers
http://www.thegoodscentscompany.com/data/rw1000251.html

Join current perfume bloggers. However, they might only know what they are told by perfumers.

https://www.fragrantica.com/news/Best-in-Show-Aldehyde-Perfumes-2020--13207.html

It stands to reason you can make perfumes like your great ancestors did and only use base oils, essential oils and floral water reasonably safely. Or you can become very thirsty for knowledge and buy Aldehydes to add, then go further and study all the chemistry of plants, their carbon chains and create. Among some of my readers there is either an accident or a very smart person about to create and market the worlds next all natural perfectly safe perfume. A little aldehyde science read:-

https://www.jlr.org/content/13/4/491.full.pdf

Tincture

In chemistry, a **tincture** is a solution that has ethanol as its solvent. In herbal **medicine**, alcoholic **tinctures** are made with various ethanol concentrations, 20% being the most common. Tinctures are not suitable for perfume making. However, you can make a perfume first then add to a tincture.

Essential Oil Study-

Not knowing enough about essential oils their effects and contra-indications is dangerous. It is best to start a perfume business after you have purchased at least 12 essential oil and have studied those oils well.

Then add more to your stock list a few at a time and study them. You should always ask your supplier of the essential oils for the data sheet for each oil. It must list all the chemicals in that oil.

Not keeping records is a dangerous mistake.

You should keep copies of all technical data on every product you use. With dates, when it arrives you need to give it a product code. See keeping a diary and Compound list.

Not Studying Absolutes

and their effects on peoples health is also dangerous. Stick to simple mixtures and you will reap the rewards. Or study hard and know exactly what you are doing and why.

Absolutes in demand include rose, jasmine, tuberose, jonquil, ylang-ylang, mimosa, boronia, lavender, lavandin, geranium, clary sage, violet, oak moss, tonka bean. Violet and Oak moss are now on the perfumers banned list in natural form.

My choice is geranium and lavender as my absolute

DIY Signature Perfume Creating

As an example of what to study about absolutes I have given you an outline of Tonka Bean. This info on Tonka Bean is from http://www.seoc.com.au/product.asp?pID=6808&cID=231

Tonka Bean
Method of extraction: Solvent extracted
Plant part: Beans

Extra Info: An Absolute may come in the form of either a solid perfume, a semi-solid or a highly viscous liquid. It is the material extracted from the plant by way of solvent extraction. This produces a concrete which is made up of fats, waxes, essential oils & other plant matter. The Absolute is then extracted from the concrete by way of using ethanol (alcohol) as a solvent.

Waxes
Such as frankincense need heating or they will not blend. But you can buy Frankincense already heated into a liquid added to Jojoba oil.
You can also warm up a cup of rice and sit the Essential oil bottle in the warm rice. Be careful though essential oils do not like heat.

Formulating Tips:
Because frankincense contains a high percentage of waxy resins it is very likely that it won't fully dissolve straight into base oils or alcohol when making a perfume blend. There are many ways around this including adding more frankincense than you need and then filtering off the un-dissolved portion to re-cycle in a wax-based product such as a balm or butter. Otherwise, it is sometimes possible to increase the solubility by gentle heating and/ or adding other chemically similar ingredients such as rose geranium to it to help break up the waxes.

However, if you purchase it as an essential oil blend in Jojoba oil it has already been heat treated and will pour from the dripolator easily. I myself like it in a bottle with an eyedropper and request same from my supplier.

Caution: Nontoxic, non-irritant and non-sensitising. Avoid during pregnancy.

How Long Will A Fragrance Last

**A Perfume Last Only As Long As
Its Designed To Last.**
We will talk about this more in the section called "Shelf-Life".

The strength of a perfume comes from the strength of the individual aromas used to make the perfume.

It is not possible to make an aroma chemical stronger than it is by adding all sorts of additive.

The aroma chemicals are simply as strong as each chemical naturally is.

Most people hope that adding a perfume fixative will address the problem of a short-lived perfume.
I like to add my perfume to my petticoat or a timber necklace. Yet on the days I do not do this people ofter remark they love my fragrance many hours after I can no longer smell it.

Unfortunately, there is not a fixative that can be added to a perfume giving it the staying power most people wish for. Adding fixatives only work to a certain point.

A long-lasting perfume is in the actual formula of a perfume. Choosing long-lasting raw materials is the ONLY way to have a long-lasting perfume.

Fixatives aromas like the Violet, Citrus and Orris fixative, are best if used as the actual base of the perfume along with other long-lasting aromas. But tall bar the citrus oils will render the perfume an unnatural perfume, just like all other perfumes in the stores.

Most of the raw aroma chemicals have longevity in hours stated in the aroma description. Look for 250 to 400 -hour longevity. The most common characteristic of a long-lasting material is thick, gooey and heavy. Some are sticky or solid. Usually the more volatile a chemical the quicker it dissipates. Such as your high notes which are actually the big attraction aromas.

There are challenges in creating fresh light perfumes with heavy rich base notes. This is when the use of ionones is a good choice the violet fixative and citrus fixative base are great choices for fresh light floral or citrus perfumes. Here is a great guide to the Ionones. However violet is now on the banned list and you will need to buy a synthetic alternative. **Ionones** are aroma compounds found in a variety of essential oils, including rose oil. β-**Ionone** is a significant contributor to the aroma of roses, despite its relatively low concentration, and is an important fragrance chemical used in perfumery. The **Ionones** are derived from the degradation of carotenoids. Lemon grass also has natural ionone.

Ionones (Pronounced Ahy-ah-nohns) a light-yellow to colorless, slightly water-soluble liquid that is either one or a mixture of two unsaturated ketones having the formula $C_{13}H_{20}O$, used chiefly in perfumery.

However, most Ionones are not suitable for the perfumer deciding to be all natural or productions of healing perfumes. Eucalyptus Dives is from the eucalyptus tree not the herb & it is not safe for natural perfumes..

http://www.leffingwell.com/chirality/ionone_irone.htm

Have a look at the aroma profile associated with each raw perfume ingredient. This will help you understand how the aroma will behave on the skin. Using aromas with greater longevity will assure a long-lasting perfume. The more you use in a formula the better. This is also where musk aromas come in handy.

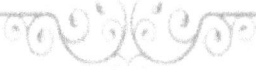

Bottles

You will need to source some bottles.

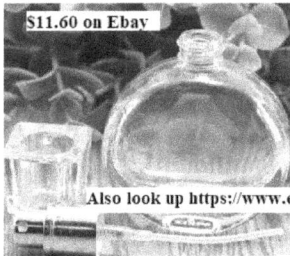

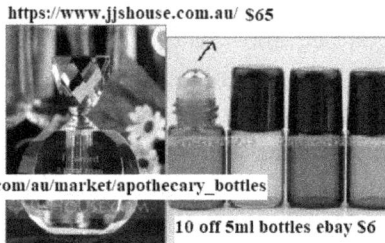

$11.60 on Ebay

https://www.jjshouse.com.au/ $65

Also look up https://www.etsy.com/au/market/apothecary_bottles

10 off 5ml bottles ebay $6

Sorry this picture is not clear but the addresses have been added below

Signature style bottle research can be very time consuming but the most important decision you need to make here is how well will it **seal** the contents when traveling. I have only ever made signature perfumes for friends and family which I deliver personally to them therefore, I am not going to be very helpful when it comes to sourcing fancy bottles that travel well. I have added a few I found this week but have not tested their ability to travel. Pictured above look for manufacturers with a good reputation.
http://www.sheleeglass.com/a/100ml_glass_bottle/apple%20shaped%20perfume%20bottle.html

Email: xuelee8884@gmail.com,

DIY Signature Perfume Creating

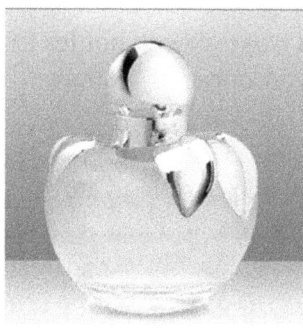

Siginture Perfume Bottles

100ml apple shaped glass perfume bottle with metal cap

Specifications of glass perfume bottle:

1, Material:Glass
    cap material: Metal

2,Capacity:100ml

3, Post processing:Printing logo, frost, hot stamping, hand polishing, decals,spraying, coating, metalization, flocking, laser engraving, laser cutting etc.

Check more information about 100ml glass perfume bottles, please feel free to contact us or leave your email, we will contact you as soon as possible.

Therapeutic Glass Bottles

My therapeutic bottles 1980s to 1990s I always got from the Bottle People In Sydney. But you can now get them online and do not need to spend $500 as a base order.

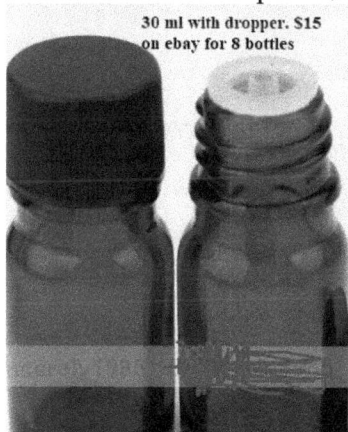

30 ml with dropper. $15 on ebay for 8 bottles

Bottles For Testing Perfume Mix.

30 ml with eyedropper 8 off on ebay $30

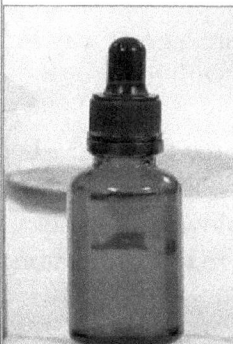

Other Bottle Choices

First, I am no pro at taking photos. I do apologise about the photos they do not reproduce well I take them with my Samsung s10 mobile phone. Some are shots I get off suppliers' web pages. I always put their website details in. You will get what I am trying to tell you easier if I add a photo.

Be Marvelously Alive.

You can purchase blue, green or brown narrow neck bottles in many sizes with either dripolators or eyedropper as well as spray atomizers.

Natural perfumes need to be in a narrow neck bottle to stop the oils from going rancid.

You can purchase blue, green or brown narrow neck bottles in many sizes with either dripolators or eyedropper as well as spray atomizers.

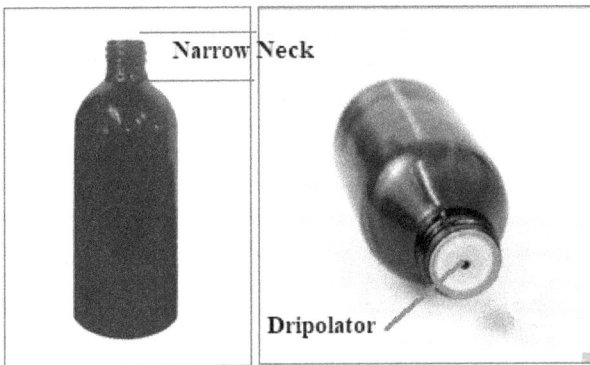

Narrow Neck

Dripolator

Roll-on bottles are a great way for a client to carry her perfume around with her.

These ones I source from New Directions.
Not only do dripolators come in slow and fast drips, some oils are thicker and slow to drop out. Also, eyedroppers give different drop size to a dripolator.

12ml Black Roll On Bottle with Stainless Steel Roll

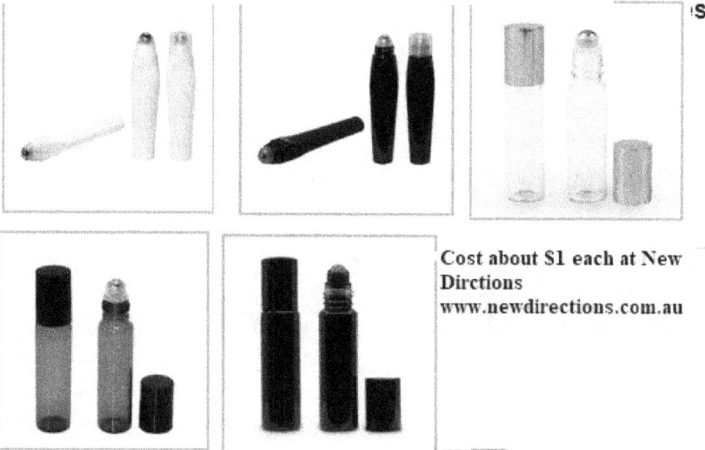

's

Cost about $1 each at New
Dirctions
www.newdirections.com.au

Where to fill Bottle too

Height: 85mm   Example of 30ml bottle

Diameter: 31.8mm

Drawing (dimensions are in millimetres):

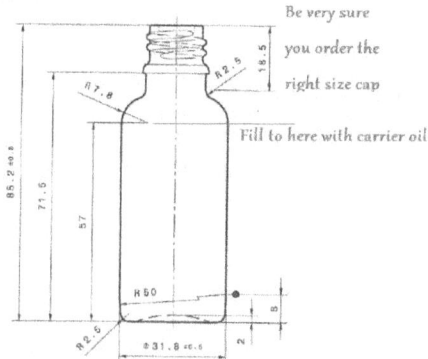

Be very sure
you order the
right size cap

Fill to here with carrier oil

Do not over fill your bottle and the fill will depend on the use of a dripolator or an eyedropper. For a dripolator you can fill a little higher that the mark in this diagram.

Pressure Seal Bottle Tops

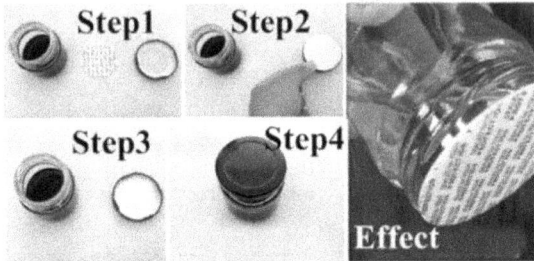

How to use

Step1   Step2

Step3   Step4

Effect

20mm/ 24mm/ 28mm/ 38mm/ 63mm/
61.5mm/ 71.5mm/ 81.5mm/ 95mm **size**

for your choice

Pressure seals can be purchased on eBay. They are
very easy to apply. They are a must do. If you do not
seal your bottle the use by date will be shorter and you
will not successfully be able to send in the post.

1. Just place on the top of the bottle press down.

2. Wait about 20 minutes then carefully screw down the
   cap

3. In 24 hours, you have a great seal. Do not post to
   anyone before the 24 hours period as it takes that long
   for the glue to set.

DIY Signature Perfume Creating

Heat Shrink

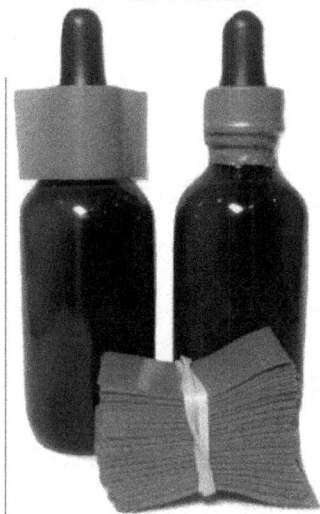

As a second line of defence I heat wrap the bottles and jars.

This is a very professional look. It is a sleeve you place over the top of the bottle and heat with your hair drying gun. They come in clear plus a variety of colours.

Test Bottles –
For Making Your Signatures- Test Fragrances.

When testing during this course it might be best to have a few clear glass bottles to mix your signatures in. This way you will see how well they are blending with your carriers. Then place them in a narrow neck Brown, amber, green, red or blue glass bottle

Essential oils are volatile liquids light turns the odour molecules rancid very quickly even when inside a air tight container.
For this reason you will need to transfer the mixtures you are happy with into a dark narrow neck bottle.

Why Natural Is Best

Start with 30 or 50 ml clear glass bottles. The quantity will depend on how many of each test signatures you are going to make in each category.

Such as
1. Oriental
2. Woody
3. Floral
4. Masculine
5. Musk *(See my notes on Mask)*

Droppers

Suppliers usually state: From time to time our packaging dimensions change depending on where we source our stock so please check with an actual bottle before committing to labels. Samples are available and single bottles can be purchased for this purpose.

This dripolator fits **Amber** bottles with a 20mm neck.
Height: 18mm
Diameter: 14.5mm
Material: Polypropylene (PP)
Drawing (dimensions are in millimeters):

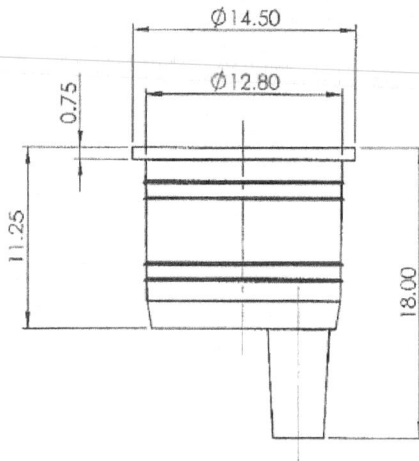

WARNING: Also when ordering bottles you need to be certain that the dripolator and cap are the same size and are designed for that particular bottle.

Droppers come in different types such as a fast drop and a slow drop. I once upon a time bought all slow droppers for my bottles and as some oils are thicker than others, I had to stand there with the bottle waiting for each drop to come out ever so slowly.

Another time I went to a demonstration day on essential oils at a doTerra demonstration day. I picked up a bottle of their oil to put on a test strip and it flowed out like it was a wide mouth jar of water. I felt so embarrassed as it was one of their most expensive oils. But for such a large company not to know the difference was interesting.

Also, the oil was not pure as they so claimed. When on the strip I noticed a ring of yellow around the edge of the wet area. The type of oil I was testing should not have done that.

Most pure essential oil can be tested by putting 1 drop onto white paper when it dries there should be no sign of the oil. If you can see a mark then it may have something added to it. *This cannot be a true test with waxy oil. With thick waxy oil you can warm up a cup of rice and sit the Essential oil bottle in the warm rice. Be careful though essential oils do not like heat.*

Air Bubbles & Dripolators

All oils are different in thickness, and will behave differently, and any aromatherapist or perfume makers - needs to respect that and take it into account when trying to carefully measure their oils. Try not to get into the habit of completely upending your bottles, or shaking them to release the oil: oils from different companies will often have different dripolator inserts and so will of course behave differently. Tilt the bottle very gently if you're unsure if it's going to pour too quickly.
 Some essential oil companies use different rate flow dripolators for the different thickness of oils and some do not. The most common problem for a blockage or other issue in an AG (Aromatherapy Grade) essential oil bottle is an **air bubble** stuck in the dripolator insert. This is primarily because oils are sent to you via Post, via road via air or in a cargo container on a ship. Travelling on their way to you, with the bottles on their side and bumping about the whole time, can easily cause an air bubble to catch in the head of the dripolator. - but usually easily fixed.

Dripolators are inserted into the rim of the bottle. Their main function is to stop oxygen from entering the bottle and to act as a **flow restrictor:** if a child or pet was to accidentally grab a potentially toxic bottle of oil, having a flow restrictor in the rim of the bottle means that they can't just upend the contents into their mouth. This is why it's a legal requirement to include dripolators in bottles of oil of a certain size and upwards - it's a safety measure.

 A good point to remember if you are producing natural perfumes.

When using a signature (fancy) style bottle - a warning must be inside the box telling people to keep out of reach of children and pets.

These flow restrictors have been designed with a central nozzle where the oil pours out, and a tiny air intake hole

By Robyn Ji Smith   page. 60

around the inside of the rim (some types have more than one intake hole). If either of those holes gets an air bubble - whether it's because it's a new bottle that hasn't been used, perhaps you're moving your oils around a lot, they haven't been used for a while.

Quick fix - just tap the bottle on a solid surface a couple of times. More often than not this will dislodge the bubble and the bottle will be ready to go. If not, you can also try inserting a pin into either of the two holes, or holding a tissue against the dripolator to suck the oil/bubble through. *This cannot be a true test with waxy oil.* **With thick waxy oil** y*ou can warm up a cup of rice and sit the Essential oil bottle in the warm rice. Be careful though essential oils do not like heat.* If your bottle is pouring too quickly, rather than being clogged as such, these same methods can also help sort the problem for you.

Thicker / Thinner Oils
The thing to be aware of, though, is that the holes in these dripolators are generally a standard size that doesn't take into account the fact that oils vary greatly in thinness or thickness of the liquid, so with the extremes you are going to find that they might behave differently depending on the viscosity of the oil.

Thicker Oil, such as Patchouli or Myrrh, may actually be quite viscous and thick, pure Rose Absolutes, will even solidify in colder weather There's usually not much you can do to get these to drip quickly - try warming the bottle in your hand or pocket for a while. You do not want it to warm up too much as excessive heat is damaging to essential oils).

Thinner Oils, such as Eucalyptus or Lemon, run much quicker and if you have a blockage that suddenly clears then they will absolutely pour out - which is probably what you **don't** want. An easy trick is to make a habit of tapping your bottle on a hard surface before you invert it to drip is a great habit.

If you're still finding that your bottle pours too quickly, try tilting it by 45 degrees. Or sitting the bottle in warm not hot rice for just a minute.

Eyedroppers

Eyedroppers are far easier to use but often leave the essential oil in the bottle exposed to the air.

Study First -
Before The Alure To Create Captivates You

Read this entire book and do your research. A perfume chemist studies for many years before he can begin. You grabbed this book and want to start now. I get that. But I am sure most of you are wanting to go natural.

It is important to understand that a natural fragrance anyone can make but to sell it to others there are laws to protect the public and you will be best advised to know those laws and the safety requirements.

I am also assuming you have little formal training in perfumery or non. Blending for yourself carries no rules or government standards to worry about.

Don't worry, if you strike gold and blend a perfume that many adore - you can have a cosmetic chemist (for a fee) sign off on your work. Document your mixture well just in case you want to sell to multitudes.

Therefore, we will cover documenting your blend in this book. The more documentation you supply to the chemist the less expensive he will be

All natural perfumes do not need a chemist to sign off on your work. If you are going to stick to all natural with a good contra-indication leaflet added to the box then you will find this book a big help.

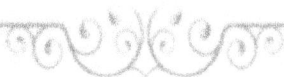

Carrier Oil

IN ESSENCE..."Carrier Oil" is a term given to base oils that dilute essential oils before topical application, as the latter (essential oils) are far too potent to apply directly to the skin.

Despite also being referred to as vegetable oils, not all Carrier Oils are derived from vegetables; many are pressed from seeds, nuts, or kernels.

Carrier Oils are also referred to as "fixed oils," due to the fact that they do not quickly evaporate from the skin's surface and remain "fixed" on the skin. They also work there way down through the skin carrying the essential oils with them into the blood stream and into the organs within 20 minutes.

A Carrier Oil is a vital aspect of an aromatherapy massage or a natural cosmetic, as it can affect the benefits and usefulness of the essential oils and the colour, scent, therapeutic properties, and shelf life of the final product, respectively.

Each Carrier Oil is comprised of different components that exhibit distinct characteristics, such as colour, viscosity, and penetration speed, while offering therapeutic properties.

1. Olive Oil
2. Grapeseed Oil
3. Jojoba Oil (*Note is a liquid wax.*)

Why Natural Is Best

4. Apricot Kernel Oil
5. Almond Oil
6. Avocado Oil
7. Coconut Oil
8. Coconut Fractionated Oil

Note Fractionated Coconut Oil is Rancid Resistant. Widely used in cosmetic and perfume as an oil diluent. Fractionated coconut oil may not be compatible with perfumers alcohol. It will separate. However, can safely be used as a base oil in perfume.

Apricot Oil

Description: Apricot Oil is good for all skin types. It is very rich and nourishing - particularly in vitamin A.
Colour: Slight Yellow
Aromatic Description: Apricot oil has very little scent characteristic of most carrier oils

Common Uses: Apricot Kernel is a very popular oil and is suitable for manufacturers, aromatherapists and massage therapists.
Consistency: Typical and Characteristic of Carrier Oils.
Absorption: Absorbs into skin quickly
Shelf life: Apricot oil is slow to go rancid; users can expect a shelf life of 6 Months to 1 Year with proper storage conditions (cool, out of direct sunlight). **Refrigeration after opening is recommended, and must be stated in you boxed instruction**

Almond Oil

Ingredients: Prunis Amygdalus Dulcis Oil
Sweet Almond is an excellent emollient and is known for its ability to soften and re-condition the skin. It is rich in proteins and Vitamin D, and is considered extremely nourishing - particularly when used regularly.

Massage therapists should note that it can stain sheets.

Botanical name: Prunus dulcis
Extraction method: Cold pressed
Common uses: Sweet Almond is a very popular, all-purpose carrier oil. It is used by manufacturers, Aromatherapists, and massage therapists.

Consistency: Typical and characteristic of carrier oils.
Absorption: Absorbs into skin at average speed, slight oil feeling left on skin.

Avocado Oil

Ingredients: Persea Gratissima Oil * * Denotes Certified Organic
Botanical Name: Persea americana
Extraction Method: Cold Pressed
Description: Avocado contains Vitamins A, B1, B2, D, E, and Beta carotene. It is classified as a monosaturated oil. It is best suited for dry skin conditions in topical applications.
Colour: Yellow/Green to Green/Brown depending upon the Lot. Avocado may go cloudy in low temperatures but will return to normal.
Aromatic Description: Avocado has very little scent characteristic of most carrier oils
Common Uses: Small amounts of Avocado Oil is typically added to other carrier oils in order to enrich protein and vitamin content. It is used predominantly by manufacturers (particularly great in soaps, lotions and creams) and massage therapists.
Consistency: Typical but slightly thicker than most Carrier Oils.
Absorption: Avocado will leave a sticky, waxy feel if applied topically to large areas of skin
Shelf life: Avocado oil is slow to go rancid; users can expect a shelf life of 9 Months to well

over 1 Year with proper storage conditions (cool, out of direct sunlight). Refrigeration after opening is recommended.

As a carrier oil you would only use 5% and is not suitable as a perfume base oil.

Coconut Oil

Botanical Name: Prunus armeniaca
Extraction Method: Cold Pressed
Ingredients: Cocos Nucifera Oil * * Denotes Certified Organic
Botanical Name: Cocos nucifera
Extraction Method: Cold Pressed
Description: Coconut oil is solid at room temperature. It is used to create a barrier on the skin. It is also the preferred oil for high quality cold process soapers.
Colour: White to off white
Aromatic Description: Coconut has a very slight coconut scent, but is generally considered odourless
Common Uses: Coconut is the preferred oil for both the soap making and cosmetic manufacturing industries.
Consistency: Solid at room temperatures. Gentle heating is required.
Absorption: Coconut creates an oily, protective barrier on the skin.
Shelf life: Coconut oil is slow to go rancid; users can expect a minimum shelf life of 6
months, but much longer with proper storage conditions (cool, out of direct sunlight). Refrigeration after opening is recommended.
Cautions: Direct application to the face with Coconut should be avoided because of possible allergic reactions.
Note: Coconut oil is solid at room temperature, however gentle heating will allow it to liquefy.

DIY Signature Perfume Creating

Fractionated Coconut Oil

Botanical Name: Cocos nucifera
Plant Part: Fruit
Extraction Method: Heat Processed
Description: Coconut Fractionated (MCT) Oil is a 60/40 grade oil that is a liquid at room temperature. It differs from Regular Coconut Oil in that it is produced by heat rather than cold pressing. Many consider it to be very comparable to the characteristics of human skin. It is also used on oily skin as it will not clog pores. It can also be used as a treatment to condition dull or dry hair.
Colour: Clear to Pale yellow
Aromatic Description: Fractionated Coconut has no scent characteristic of most carrier oils
Common Uses: Fractionated coconut is used almost exclusively by cosmetic manufacturers.
Consistency: Typical and Characteristic of Carrier Oils.
Absorption: Fractionated Coconut produces a barrier on the skin, but will not clog pores.
Shelf life: Fractionated Coconut oil is very slow to go rancid; users can expect a minimum shelf life of 6 months, but much longer with proper storage conditions (cool, keep out of direct sunlight). Refrigeration after opening is recommended.
Cautions: Allergic reactions to this oil is a possibility, though less so than regular coconut
Grapeseed Oil
Ingredients: Vitis Vinifera Seed Oil * * Denotes Certified Organic
Extraction Method: Cold Pressed
Aroma: This oil can have a slightly vinegar-like aroma. May not be suitable for all perfume blends.
Colour: Light to mid yellow with a green tinge.
Benefits: An economical oil with mildly astringent properties which make this suitable for all but the very driest skin types. The low level of free oleic acid makes this quite a mild oil which gives it a low irritancy potential. This is a high shine oil that has a medium to long rub-in time making it especially suitable for hair products and colour cosmetics.

Jojoba Oil

Jojoba carrier oil works well for making perfume.
It moisturizes the skin, absorbs quickly without leaving a
greasy effect.

Jojoba oil is odorless and colourless.
Jojoba is a shrub that grows in dry regions of northern Mexico
and the southwestern US. The seeds of the jojoba plant
incorporate as much as 60% of their weight in oil. The oil is
best isolated by cold pressing of the seeds. The raw extract is
called "jojoba wax," and removing the glycerine leaves jojoba
oil.

- Jojoba oil has many uses: moisturizer, hair care
  products
- anti-aging creams, softening cuticles, restoring natural
  skin oil balance
- removing makeup
- acne treatment and prevention
- Jojoba oil mixed with essential oils is perfect, it will
  give any perfume recipe that little extra touch.

Olive Oil

Description: Olive is an extremely versatile oil. It is a
favourite on both dry and irritated skin.
Colour: Yellow with Green Tones
Aromatic Description: Olive Oil has an appealing odour, but
an odour that can influence essential oils if in a blend.
Common Uses: Olive Oil can be used for any application,
though it may not be a preferred choice in any particular
category.
Consistency: Typical and Characteristic of Carrier Oils.
Absorption: Olive Oil will leave an oily feeling on the skin.
But has many healing properties.
Shelf life: Olive oil is slow to go rancid; users can expect a
shelf life of 6 Months to 1 year with proper storage conditions

(cool, out of direct sunlight). Refrigeration after opening is recommended.

Other Carries For Essential Oils

1. Aloe Vera Gel
2. Shea Butter
3. Talc
4. Wool Fat

I would like to add at this point that cream perfumes and Talc work well as a perfume base. How much of the perfume compound, you mix into the talc or cream can be very tricky and a little dangerous. There are many terms used and you need to read this section with care. We are bordering on medicinal and that comes with responsibilities that follow laws. Sure, you can make a lip balm without being a certified Aromatherapist or healer but to add a perfume compound to lip balms and such is unkind and unlawful.

Stick to the blending table quantities.

Balms
Balms are considered ointments.

Emulsifiers
Commonly used products in aromatherapy as Emulsifiers include but are not limited to:-
- PEG-7 Glyceryl Cocoate (a coconut oilbased emulsifier),
- perfumers alcohol,
- Polysorbate 20, 60 or 80,
- Turkey Red Sulphated Castor oil,
- Bees wax, to name a few.
- Emulsifiers will help the essential oils to blend with your water based products.

Emollients

Emollients are ingredients like plant oils, bees wax, mineral oil, shea butter, tonka bean butter, cocoa butter, petrolatum, and fatty acids (animal oils, including emu, mink, and lanolin, the latter probably the one ingredient that is most like our own skin's oil).

At this point I do want to talk a little about lanolin, because it is very close in structure to human skin. Yes, it is an animal by product. But there are times when it will assist people with skin issues and is far better than steroids.

You can add it to other products and oils to make a wax perfume. But you cannot add a perfume compound to it and call it a skin repairer, unless you are a qualified healer.

The Emollient That Cured Me

I myself had an allergic reaction to high blood pressure tablets, I am in my 70s. What happened - my skin suddenly became very dry and annoyingly itchy with a prickly heat sensation.

I had no idea it was the tablets. This was a very uncomfortable situation. The itch was all over my body including my scalp, my skin was extremely dry and brittle. No matter what blends I made and applied, the relief was only for about 30 to 70 minutes. This horrible annoying nerve-racking skin situation went on for almost a year. Finally, I talked to my GP about it and she sent me to a dermatologist. The creams he recommended did not help at all.

When my skin test came back all they could tell me was it was a drug related rash. As I have never taken drugs and drink alcohol only on an odd occasion I was instantly confused.

Then I thought, Oh, I am taking blood pressure tablets. I sent the dermatologist a message that I needed to speak with him. We chatted for a while and talked about the oils I use and he suggested I research the chemical compound of each oil and stop taking the blood pressure tablets for a few weeks. I did stop the tablets and the itch dwindled within days.

My skin on the other hand had not improved. Extremely dry skin is very irritating. My normal olive oil base was not emollient enough to repair my damaged skin.

My Bichon Frise (Dog) after he turned 12 his skin became very dry and sensitive and he would nibble at his skin and make it bleed. For him I used Rose geranium and lavender in Olive oil. It healed him very quickly but for me it did not improve my skin irritation. I made skin peels and skin scrubs but as quick as I would get rid of the top layers of dead skin I would bleed. My skin was dry right down as far as the subcutaneous tissue and increasing my Olive Oil intake was not working quickly enough.

So here is what I did and got results within 3 days.

Step one
In one 50gram jar of anhydrous wool fat I Removed some of the wool fat from the jar. added
20ml olive oil
10 drops of Rose Geranium
5 drops of Clarysage
5 drops Lavender
Put the lid on the jar and gently warmed it in a saucepan of warm water on a low heat.
Stirred with a glass stick.
Massaged into my entire body
Wrapped myself in glad wrap (*plastic food wrap*)
After one hour removed the plastic wrap
Lathered my body with pure soap and water

Used bicarbonate of soda as my exfoliant
Took a shower and shampooed my hair.

Step two
In a750ml bottle of olive oil I added
30 drops of Rose Geranium
25 drops of Clarysage
25 drops Lavender
5 drops Eucalyptus
Gave bottle a shake.
After my shower I applied this oil
Then applied again A few hours later.

Step three
Every morning and night
I had a tablespoon of Bicarbonate of soda in water
Followed by a hot lemon drink with half a lemon squeezed
into a cup added 1 teaspoon of honey and boiling water.

I also drank half a cup of virgin olive oil.

On day four I did not need the wool-fat mix.

I religiously did steps two and three for one month.
With all that said, I am a lover of wool fat and lanolin in some situations. Therefore, I am suggesting you make your cream perfume with a wool fat base if you have dry aging skin.

Just recently I had to have some anti biotics and although I explained to the specialist that I am allergic to most medications they insisted I take them. They researched what kind I maybe able to tolerate. But still my dry skin and itch came back within 4 days. I stopped taking them straight away and went back to steps one to three for a few days and I am all good again.

My skin will never look as good as it did before this ordeal as I have scars but hey, I am in my seventies so nothing looks as good as it once did. LOL.

I pray my storey may help someone else with dry cracked skin. If you see an elderly person with dry bleeding skin you will now know how to help them. But you cannot add a perfume compound of essential oils to the base oil.

Now you know why I as a aromatherapist who should only be giving you mixtures that are all animal free. I advocate the use sometimes of other products. I am old and come from a family natural cure healers.

At this point you may think this was an over kill but my nervous system had also gone haywire due to the constant itch. You sometime have to go that extra mile.

Balms, Salves and Ointments

You may consider adding a perfume signature to other base products and should understand there are many names you can call these items. But a balm, slave, liniment fragrant cream or liquid used to heal or soothe the skin and such, should not be considered as terms for creamy waxy product that you add a signature perfume compound to. Unless you are a Certified Healer and are going to have the end product registered with TGA

Keep a lid on your growth.
We are in this book designing natural perfumes with the idea that you may want to expand into alcohol-based perfumes, natural cream perfumes and perfumed talc.

Not even a lip balm or lip gloss as these are also considered to be a healing product and a perfume compound has not been designed with healing purposes in mind. However, a blend or compound can be mixed

But that method has not been included in this book. Why not, you might ask? Because in 50 odd years of teaching I have found one module at time, well learned, works best.

Why Natural Is Best

Similar Terms:	Terms you can use
ointment	no
lotion	Yes
cream	Yes
salve	No
liniment	No
embrocation	No
rub	No
gel	Yes
emollient	Yes
unguent	No
balsam	Yes
moisturizer	Yes
pomade	Yes
pomatum	No
demulcent	No
humectant	Yes
unction	No
Opposite:	
astringent	Yes
irritant	Yes

Hydrosols

Which brings me to another term. Hydrosols
Hydrosols are made from the water left in the distil after
essential oils have been extracted. They are also known as
floral waters.

Although essential oils have been distilled to make floral
waters -essential oil will not dissolve and become miscible in
floral waters.

They have all the benefits of the essential oil they were
derived from, but without the potency of the essential oil
which renders them safe to use straight from the bottle.

They can be used in alcohol based perfumes in place of water.

A hydrosol can be packaged as a spritz in a clear glass bottle
as it is not volatile like its mother (Essential Oils)

Remember though that essential oils cannot be added to skin
products when a hydrosol is the base.

Infused Oil

An infused oil, also referred to as a macerated oil, consists of a carrier oil that has been permeated ("infused" or "macerated") with one or more herbs. The benefit to using an infused oil as opposed to a plain carrier oil is that the infused oil will contain the properties of both the carrier oil and the herbs that were infused into the oil.

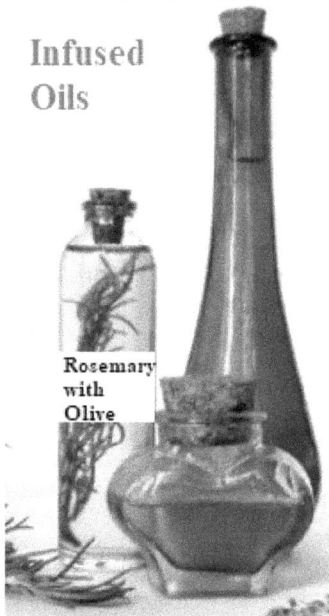

Infused
Oils

Rosemary
with
Olive

Infused oils are great for both cooking and adding to a base oil in perfume making.

Some plants do not have much essential oil contained in them, and in those cases, it is rare or impossible to commercially find an essential oil for that plant species. Infusing the herb into a carrier oil, however, can be a suitable way to still use the herb for aromatherapy purposes.

I like doing this with date seeds because the essential oil is hard to find and I am never sure it is pure when purchased from suppliers I do not know. It is normally discarded but date seeds are composed of carbohydrates, dietary fiber, fat, ash and protein. Some studies have shown date seeds have defensive effect against chemically-induced liver damage and oxidative DNA damage. I also do this with Jasmin flowers because I have a vine. I use the jasmine oil in perfumes and the date seed infused oil I add to salads.

Infused oils generally have an oily feeling that varies depending on the carrier oil used. They also are not as concentrated as essential oils. Additionally, infused oils, just like carrier oils, can go rancid.

It is important that you heed the safety information and contra-indications of the herbs you choose to use in your infused oil.

How to Make an Infused Oil

The easiest way to make an infused oil is by the use of a crock pot with a very low heat setting. Since the infused oil must be gently heated, it is essential that your crock pot does not overheat the oil. Do not use a crock pot that only has one heat setting as that crock pot most likely will overheat the oils.

Add 50 milliliters (2 ounces) of your chosen carrier oil and half kilo of dried herbs (if you use fresh herbs, double the amount of herbs used) to your spotlessly-clean crock pot and stir well.

Turn your crock pot to the lowest heat setting.

Allow to heat on the lowest setting for two hours, stirring every 10-15 minutes (setting a timer to remind you to stir is important). After two hours, carefully strain the oil by using unbleached muslin, gauze or coffee filters. You should strain the oil at least twice. If any herbs remain in the infused oil, the oil can go rancid.

Essential Oil Study

You need to study essential oils. For each oil you add to your kit, you need to know all about it.

If you are going to make natural perfumes for yourself and family, follow my blending instructions and the contra-indication list under the headings in this book.
Pages 102 to 107 "Blending Table" and "Blending Table Chart"

If you follow those instruction well, you will not actually need to know much about the oils, just the smell must be to your liking.

However, if you are going to blend to sell you better know what you are doing and know the oils you use well.

Let us look at "Thyme" at one of the suppliers I have used for the past 30 odd years. New Directions. Springfields have been around for a long time actually longer than new directions but their website is not as informative as it could be. They have a Thyme oil 17ml for $33 and a Red Thyme oil for $12.10 The one for $33 is a certified therapeutic oil.

I always go for oils with a certificate but it depends on you, your purse strings and how passionate you are about the quality.

On New Direction site they have info about each oil but I do not like their heading on safety. Or cautions.

17 ml Thyme Red Essential Oil

Product number: OE17THYMRED

AU$12.10

1

PRODUCT DESCRIPTION

Ingredients: Thymus Vulgaris Flower/Leaf Oil
Botanical name: Thymus vulgaris L.

Common name: Red Thyme

Plant part: Flowering stem with leaves

Extraction method: Steam distilled

Common uses: Thyme oil has traditionally been used to help relieve gout, arthritis and rheumatic pain.

Note: Top

Strength of aroma: Strong

Aromatic scent: Warm, Spicy-herbaceous aroma

Cautions: Non-toxic and non-irritating. Possible sensitiser in some individuals. Avoid during pregnancy.

17 ml Thyme Certified Organic Oil - ACO 10282P

Product number: OC17THYM

AU$33.00

1

PRODUCT DESCRIPTION

Ingredients: Thymus Vulgaris Oil * * Denotes Certified Organic
Botanical name: Thymus vulgaris

Common name: White Thyme

Plant part: Leaves

Extraction method: Steam distilled

Common uses: Thyme oil has traditionally been used to help relieve gout, arthritis and rheumatic pain.

Note: Top

Strength of aroma: Strong

Aromatic scent: Warm, Spicy-herbaceous aroma

Cautions: Non-toxic and non-irritating. Possible sensitiser in some individuals. Avoid during pregnancy.

Certification: Australian Certified Organic

Why Natural Is Best

Thyme oil blends well with Bergamot, Grapefruit, Lavender, Rosemary, Oregano, and Melaleuca (Tea Tree) essential oils.

Red Thyme contains large amounts of toxic phenols, **never use thyme** in a diffuser, nor smell therapy, while pregnant, breast feeding or if you have a weak heat.

White thyme is often adulterated.

Lemon Thyme is a safer alternative because of the linalool properties in structure and is safe to use on children.

There are many benefits of Thyme.

- Antibacterial. Thymol, the most prevalent terpene in thyme oil, has antimicrobial properties. ...
- Insect Repellent. Thyme oil has been found to be quite an effective mosquito repellent. ...
- Yeast Infection. ...
- Skin Conditions. ...
- Respiratory Infections and Coughs. ...
- Alopecia/Hair Loss

All you need to know as a natural perfume designer is the contra-indications.
Then you can choose how much of that oil you should or should not add to your compound. Yet the information is out there when you research each oil in your kit, just in case you strike Gold and make a winning fragrance.

Documentation is the key because you can have a perfume chemist sign off on your work should you decide to market that perfume.

Essential Oil Aroma Substitutions

This is not a therapeutic list it is an **Aroma** substitute list for perfume making. There are also substitutes for healing oils but that is not what this book is about.

The Japanese use yuzu to make perfume, it is expensive but it is a cross between grapefruit and mandarin. Therefore, you can with experimenting make grate fragrances, without the high price tag of some ingredients.

Ylang Ylang is a fraction of the price of Jasmine because Jasmine has very tiny petals that take a long time to gather, which adds to the cost. Yet Ylang Ylang and Neroli mixed together can give a similar scent at a fraction of the price.

You need to develop a good nose and the more you smell, the more often you add just two oils together, one drop at a time, the aroma comparisons, will become mind muscles. Thus, allowing you to use substitutes for the more expensive aromas.

Use perfume tester strips or cotton wool balls or slices of timber and place one drop of two oils on two different strips, hold both strips under your nose. Smell the strips separately and decide which aroma is the strongest and maybe use less of that oil in your full compound.

You can use rose water in a alcohol blend and add rose geranium to make rose perfume without the high price tag of pure rose essential oil.

Ylang Ylang is widely used in perfumery and blends well with citrus scents like grapefruit, floral scents like lavender, and woody scents like sandalwood. Sandalwood being very expensive replace it with cedarwood.

Experiment - experiment - experiment.

Why Natural Is Best

But as my dad said to me and I have said to my children and grandchildren,

"Play Safe"

Oil Substitution List

substitutions:	
Don't Have This:	**Try This:**
Rose Otto	Rose Geranium
Tangerine	Orange
Cassia	Cinnamon
Birch	Wintergreen
Spearmint	Peppermint
Helichrysum	Frankincense
Sandalwood	Cedarwood or Amyris
Jasmine	Ylang Ylang
Clary Sage _____	Lavender
Musk	Ambrette Seeds oil Hibiscus tree pods
Myrrh	Frankincense
German Chamomile	Roman Chamomile
Angelica	Clary Sage
Balsam Fir	Blue or Black Spruce
Lemongrass	Lemon
Ginger	Cardamom
Cinnamon	Clove

Peppermint be sure you are purchasing the herb not the leaves of the eucalyptus peppermint tree.

As well as a "substitution perfume oil list", you need to develop a "Blends Well With List"

Example:
Thyme oil blends well with Bergamot, Grapefruit, Lavender, Rosemary, Oregano, and Melaleuca (Tea Tree) essential oils.

Why? Because some essential oils have chemicals that either don't like each other or too much of the same chemicals. This is not that important for perfumes mixing, but is always good to know.

Rose Geranium blends particularly well with angelica, basil, bergamot, carrot seed, cedarwood, citronella, clary sage, grapefruit, jasmine, lavender, lime, neroli, orange and rosemary.

Rose essential oil pairs well with bergamot, Roman chamomile, jasmine, geranium, ylang ylang, neroli, patchouli, vetiver, sandalwood, and frankincense essential oils.

Petitgrain essential oil is from the bitter sweet orange tree and blends well with all citrus oils. Blends well with orange, neroli, geranium, chamomile, ylang ylang, bergamot, lemon, clary sage, rosemary, lavender, jasmine, and juniper berry. Ambrette Seeds has a similar smell to the Musk of a Deer but it is not the exact perfume makers delight. However, it is natural and a Deer does not need to be killed to gain the aroma.

Essential Oil Notes

Also see heading "Essential Oil Top, Middle & Base Note List"

The Three Notes Of Essential Oils In A Perfume Are:-
1. Base Notes
2. Middle Notes
3. Top Notes.

Fragrance.

This is a very loosely used word we all need to be mindful of when buying scents/aroma products for our perfume making. The term Essential oils mostly means oils that have been extracted from plants in several ways and in different grades. There are certified essential oils for healing and essential oils that some resellers adulterate and cunningly sell as essential oils.

You need to purchase them from well-known manufacturers that are happy to give you the chemical list, or state they are certified. To purchase the uncertified is fine however, you cannot on sell your perfumes and call them pure or natural fragrances or natural perfumes.

Fragrant oils:-

Are inexpensive but have not been distilled naturally for healing purposes. They are chemically designed oils to mimic the same aroma as a natural essential oil fragrance.

Accord

The word, accord, represents two elements that combine to make a third; in one case, it's a musical composition, and in the other, a unique blended fragrance. ... They are the key to the transformation of a dull scent to a superior fragrance, and each accord represents a specific perfume family. In natural perfume formulas we call the a Compound.

DIY Signature Perfume Creating

An accord is either, your base blend and can be considered the Base blend or the finished product or the compound signature. In other words it is a mixture of several products to make a fragrance.

A Compound is a blend of all notes of essential oils. We can also call a compound a signature blend.

Even the most basic perfumes should blend three scents, or "notes." The combination of a base note, middle note and top note (added in that order) is what causes a perfume's aroma to stably change - the longer it stays on your skin.

The **base note** is added first and lingers the longest on your skin -- some essential oils can hang on for a couple of days.

Base notes are often from the woodsy family, but vanilla, vetiver and patchouli are common, too. The base oil should make up about 20 percent of your blend, but remember the chemist hired by Chole Chanel accidently added to much and that perfume has sold beyond expectations. However, as some of the ingredients are now banned the Chemist have had to make mock aromas to place in the fragrance to mimic the aroma.

The **middle note** makes up the core of your scent. It will evaporate within two to four hours, leaving the base note to react with your skin. About 50 percent.

The **top note** is what gives the first impression of your perfume, you smell it immediately. It's the last thing you add to the mix (about 30 percent) and the first scent to evaporate, usually within a couple of hours. Citrus and floral oils like orchid, chamomile and anise are popular top notes.

A few drops of a "bridge note" are sometimes added at the end to help the other notes blend together more smoothly. It's often lavender, vanilla or a very mildly scented "carrier" oil, like vitamin E or jojoba oil, that doesn't evaporate from the skin.

So you don't waste precious ingredients when you're playing around with scents, make samples. And put tags on them with a name date and number and document the mix in your perfume diary/journal.

Up until about the 1940s women did not spray perfume on their body they put it onto a cotton square or a handkerchief and placed it on their under garment.

Blend one day and smell the next. If you're happy with the combo in the morning, you'll be ready to take the next step: making the actual perfume. the two key components of a very basic perfume are oil and a diluting agent, which is a base/carrier oil for a natural blended perfume or high-proof alcohol. For a alcohol based perfume like most perfumes in stores. However, vodka and some other alcohols do not render the perfume miscible.

Adulteration of Rose Oil

It takes a large amount of rose petals to distill a small amount of essential oil. Depending on extraction method and plant species, the typical yield can be approximately 1:3,000. To mitigate the cost, some dishonest dealers will dilute rose oil with geranium (Pelargonium graveolens) or palmarosa (Cymbopogon martinii) essential oils, both of which are rich in geraniol, the main constituent of rose oil. Some of these "rose oils" are up to 90% geranium or palmarosa to 10% rose.

This is referred to as extending the rose fragrance. This may be done to compensate for chemotype, e.g. Bulgarian distilled rose oil is naturally low in phenyl ethanol, and Ukrainian or Russian rose oil is naturally high in phenyl ethanol. Pure rose oil should not be used directly on the skin, as it can cause allergic reactions such as red skin and spots.

DIY Signature Perfume Creating

If you are going to go beyond natural then this is a must read.

https://en.wikipedia.org/wiki/Phenethyl_alcohol

Sandalwood is very expensive but if you add just a few drop to a finished blend you can then add Pure Balsamic Vinegar to bring out the Balsamic aroma of sandalwood.

Secret Chemicals

A 2010 study by the Environmental Working Group revealed that many name-brand perfumes contain potentially hazardous chemicals not listed on their labels. The worst offender? I read somewhere was "Seventy Seven" by American Eagle, which contained 24 off-list ingredients.

While the perfumers in France were not the original creators of perfume, they were the geniuses that figured out a way to make the fragrances last longer than just a few minutes.

Their method was by layering the different fragrances. They started using the three layers that we now call notes.

If you've never made perfume before, you may not know the importance of using the different notes. For the best fragrances, you can't just throw together several essential oils and hope for the best. Some fragrances are stronger and longer lasting than others. Knowing what essential oils are in each note group will help you to make some beautiful and interesting creations with your perfume. Notes are what make up the difference between perfume and cologne, so we are lead to believe but I beg to differ.

I feel or like to express that a cologne is a signature/perfume compound with more alcohol and water added to it that a perfume called a "Perfume"

A perfume is the group of essential oils notes to which is added attars and absolutes are added with the alcohol.

Why Natural Is Best

Whereas, a natural perfume uses only pure essential oils, waxes, and base oils.

Perfumery is a science. Today's perfumes are made with synthetic copies of essential oils as real oils would be too expensive to use in the mass production of perfume. Perfume making is also experimental.

This is why you need to start with test bottles and less is best when it comes to the amount of oils you use. Just start with three oils in each test bottle then add, drop by drop of another oil to one test bottle.

You will find most perfumes on the market today are diluted with alcohol and water. In your own laboratory, you may also want to use oil to dilute your perfume, although using alcohol will make them last longer. As you begin to blend your fragrances, you will want to experiment with a variety of different aromas. Most perfumes fall into one of the five categories:

* Woodsy
* Floral
    1. Oriental
    2. Spicy
    3. Citrus

It takes a bit of experimenting with essential oils to get the scent that you want. Making perfume is definitely an art and, like any art, the result will depend on the time, inspiration and imagination that go in the product.

Perfume is seldom made with just one fragrance. They're usually a blend of up to three or more fragrances. These fragrances, in the perfume world, are called notes.

Perfume consists of
  • base notes,
  • middle notes

DIY Signature Perfume Creating

- top notes.

A perfume should never be decided on when a women has her periods and never during a full moon.

Perfumes are also about moods and personalities. Therefore, when deciding what perfume, you want to create - be mindful that a perfume is not an every day and night accessary.

A Frenchman called Piesse classified the odours of essential oils in the 19th century according to musical scales, and this is where the top, middle and base notes originated.

For me musically lyrically noted will be your notes forming the perfume compounds of accords. I feel that perfumes often say you are:-

- Romantically moving me
- A wild thing
- Making my heart sing
- A breath of fresh air
- Strongly willed
- Very masculine
- Naughty
- Nice
- Sweet
- A Spring time allure
- Summer
- Autumn
- Winter
- And many other moods and effects.

When a woman is in a soft fabric dress that flows as she walks or stands in a breeze and has a fragrance on that smells like spring time, she makes others feel light hearted and free.

Why Natural Is Best

When in a similar dress on a mid summer evening and her fragrance smells hearty or romantic men will be attracted to her and women feel either jealous or admire her.

A perfume must not be always just about you.

In times long gone, when a young women was going for an interview her mother would give her a pep talk, such as sit with your knees together and be up straight. Allow them to do all the talking and ask all the questions until they ask "do you have any questions".

Before leaving home her mother may say don't wear perfume today, just dust your underwear with baby talc and put bicarb on your arm pits.

The theory was not to allow all of your personality to sing out.

Musk

It is important to understand that Musk is no longer available as a natural fragrance fixative. Unless you are a qualified perfume maker. As the male Deer needs to be killed to obtain the pod and the same goes for Civet.

Photo Musk pod of the male Deer

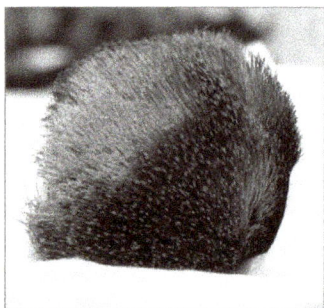

Musk is a class of aromatic substances commonly used as base notes in perfumery. They include glandular secretions from animals such as the musk deer, numerous plants emitting similar fragrances, and artificial substances with similar odours. Musk was a name originally given to a substance with a strong odour obtained from a gland of the musk deer. The substance has been used as a popular perfume fixative since ancient times and is one of the most expensive animal products in the world.

The musk pod is normally obtained by killing the male deer through traps laid in the wild. Upon drying, the reddish-brown paste inside the musk pod turns into a black granular material called "musk grain", which is then tinctured with alcohol. The aroma of the tincture gives a pleasant odour only after it is considerably diluted.

No other natural substance has such a complex aroma associated with so many contradictory descriptions; however, it is usually described abstractly as animalistic, earthy and woody or something akin to the odour of baby's skin

Some plants such as Angelica archangelica or Abelmoschus moschatus produce musky-smelling macrocyclic lactone compounds. These compounds are widely used in perfumery as substitutes for animal musk or to alter the smell of a mixture of other musks.

The plant sources include the musk flower (Mimulus moschatus) of western North America, the musk wood (Olearia argophylla) of Australia, and the musk seeds (Abelmoschus moschatus) from India.

With that said, I watched a documentary on television that was explaining that in some part of the world they need to kill wild dear as the numbers are too great.

So I can only assume we can still buy the real must oil.

Base Notes in Perfume

Base Notes

Base notes are considered the backbone of the perfume, is what the users will remember most about this particular fragrance. This scent of base notes will last the longest in the air. Examples of base notes are Vanilla, Sandalwood, Cinnamon, mosses or other woodsy scents. The middle notes are usually the inspiration for the perfume and often a floral scent such as Geranium, Honeysuckle, Jasmine, Lemongrass or Neroli. Top notes are usually the selling point for the perfume as well as the first name listed. Common top notes include Rose, Lavender, Orchid, Lemon, Bergamot or other citrus or herbal scents.

As with any good creation, it's combining the right mixture of ingredients that counts. Using notes that go well with each other will give you a beautiful fragrance you'll never tire of wearing and your friends will never tire of smelling. Your friends will constantly be asking you what you're wearing and where you got it. Imagine their surprise when you tell them it's your own creation!

One of the keys to successful perfume making is in mixing the right blend.

Don't just assume because you happen to like two different fragrances that they'll make a good mixture for perfume.

Before you waste a lot of time and money on essence oils, make some samples. Although making your own perfume is a lot cheaper than buying perfume, essence oil can get costly as well.

If you're considering blending a couple different oils together, put them on a cotton swap or perfume tester strip and let them sit overnight. In the morning, check out what they smell like and if you're pleased with the results, you have your new perfume fragrances and you're ready to start creating your own masterpiece!

Base oils (Base Notes) This will produce the scent that stays longest on the skin and for this reason it is usually added to the mixture first. Some of the fragrances with a base note include: Sandalwood, Vanilla, Patchouli, Cedarwood, Clove, Cinnamon, Mosses, Lichens, Ferns and Frankincense.

Base notes are what you smell after about 30 seconds of applying it to your skin. The based and middle notes are what make up the main fragrance of the perfume.

However, for a perfume to be successful, must have a combination of all three notes.

Middle Notes

Middle oils (also known as the Heart Notes) This also influences the smell of the perfume for quite some time, but not as long as the base notes does. Some of the fragrances with a middle note include: Lemon Grass, Geranium, Rosewood, Neroli, Jasmine, Rose, Hyacinth and Ylang-Ylang.

Middle Notes in Perfume

Middle notes are what we smell when the scent from the top notes disappears. It is generally considered as the heart of the perfume and often server to cover up any unpleasant scents that may come from the base notes. This scent often evaporates after 15 seconds.

Top Notes

Top oils (Top Notes) This is added to the mixture after the middle notes, and may then be followed by some other substance which will help to bridge the scents together. Some of the fragrances that are top note include: Orchid, Rose,

Why Natural Is Best

Bergamot, Chamomile, Lavender, Peppermint, Lemon, Orange and Lime.

Top Notes in Perfume

Top notes are the scents that you smell as soon as you apply it. If you've ever sprayed a perfume in a store, the smell you get immediately after spraying is coming from the top notes. The top notes, although they quickly evaporate, are what give us our first impression of a perfume.

Your fragrance /aroma will contain one or more from each of the above categories: base note, mid note and a top note. Some perfumers recommend using a four note, a bridge notes such as an absolute, or Lavender or Vanilla. The bridge is what will help the other three blend together well plus a base oil which is often a Vitamin E oil, Jojoba oil , Olive oil or some other oil known as a carrier oil, which you can get at a health food store or from an essential oil supplier.

The top note is the first to evaporate on your skin. It is also the first impression that you have of the fragrance. The mid note stays on a little bit more and the base note is what will remain on your skin for hours.

The base note will react with your skin to form a scent of its own. This is why no two perfumes smell exactly alike on any two people.

It is also the reason why you should test out a perfume for about a half an hour by putting a dab on your wrist, doing your shopping and then taking a sniff to see if you still like the scent.

It is very important that when you are making perfume, your mix the extracts in the above order starting with base, then the middle and finally adding the top note. Typically, you add equal amounts of each type in order to produce the right sort of perfume. Then add more of one or all three notes.

Because regular perfumes are made with synthetics, they cannot boast the phenylethylamine (natural happiness chemicals} in your brain., The nice thing about using therapeutic perfumes (Essential Oils based aromas) that you make yourself is - that the essential oils can actually help heal anything troubling you, or even give you energy, while also giving you a pleasant scent. But must be mixed with a carrier oil.

When using pure essential oils, there will be quite a difference to ratios when making perfumes, however, they are meant to be used sparingly. For instance, you will dilute the perfume signature with carrier oil or alcohol.

Your signature compound will be in a storage bottle - it is your concentrate.

You can make as little or as much as you like. It is better to start with a small quantity until you are sure it works well with the other base products you will add it too.

For Floral Notes Use
Geranium
Jasmin
Lavender
Rose,

For Woodsy Notes Use
Amyris
Frankincense
Myrrh
Sandalwood

For Oriental Notes Use
Jasmine
Ginger
Mandarin,

For Spicy Notes
Ylang Ylang.
Ginger,
Neroli,
Nutmeg.
For citrus notes
Orange,
Lemon,
Lime
Grapefruit.

Be game with your experimenting while mixing blends at home.

Perfumery is an art unto itself and takes years to practice. Perfumers today still practice this art and make scents that fail. It is all a matter of personal taste and seeing what blends well with what and a great deal to do with how people smell. Each of our DNA has a different odour. Coupled with our diet, how much alcohol a person drinks and what drugs they take.

There is an old saying that your perfume should not walk in the room before you do. You want people to remember a pleasant scent, not be overpowered by your perfume.

One nice perfume recipe that you can use is very simple and combines woodsy with oriental: However, we are not going to learn to mix perfume this way we are going to look more closely at making the test signature aromas in separate bottles then mixing the test signatures with the carrier oil.

This basic recipe for an oriental perfume is for someone to consider that does not want to go through the learning stages of mixing perfumes.

You mix this perfume at your own risk.

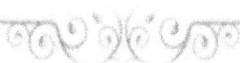

Basic Perfume Recipe – Oriental

100ml Carrier oil
10 drops Sandalwood Essential Oil (Base to Top note)
5 drops Jasmine Essential Oil (Top Note)
2-3 drops Ylang Ylang Essential Oil (Base note}
1-2 drops of Lavender. To tie the aroma molecules together.
Lavender is an equalizer.

This particular aroma is a very romantic perfume! Perfumes were commonly used as aphrodisiacs to attract a mate. This one has a unique scent with a pleasant base note, but again, perfume scents are very subjective. Be sure to experiment a little before you decide to open up your own perfumery.

In addition to being a pleasant perfume, the above aromatherapy fragrance also works to promote energy as well as assisting in creating a romantic mood. Both Jasmine and Ylang Ylang are powerful aphrodisiacs, so only use this blend with caution.

You will find the recipe listed above is also beneficial for relaxing as well. The benefits of using aromatherapy in your own perfumes are the following:

Completely natural products and non-toxic

Have healing powers as well as a pleasant fragrance

You can have a scent that no one else has (don't underestimate this one – there are people who pay plenty to create their own scent at perfumeries in Paris).

Much less expensive in the long run.

Why Natural Is Best

The disadvantages? You have to play around with scents for a little bit before you hit on what you like. Make sure that you write each ratio of every essential oil used in a particular scent. Be a document freak. Nothing can be more frustrating than actually coming up with the fragrance of your dreams and then not remembering how you ended up making it.
 Although I write the blend in my diary, I add a swing tag with a name or number to the test bottle, put a label on the bottle with the scent kind such as woody, .

A test bottle will be filled with the aromatic blend compound, and not have the fillers added such as water, base oil, alcohol or cream.

The cream is another base we will look at later. Called cream base.

Keep in mind, when making your perfume, that you can mix and match different essential oils to get the scent that you want. You can add as many as your heart desires. But do it one drop at a time. Or you can simply add one essential oil to alcohol and add a flowered water.

The purpose of using the specific notes is to ensure you have a fragrance that's not only appealing but one that lasts as well. **A natural perfume artisan** will also strive to cause no harm to a persons skin, organs of their body, or their unborn child.

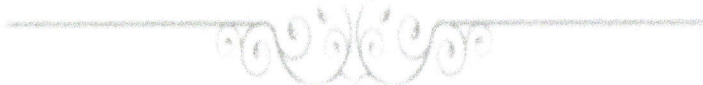

Essential Oil Top, Middle & Base Note List

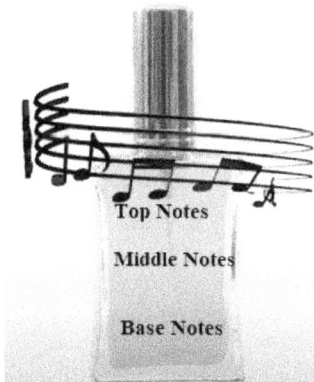

The following essential oils are considered

Top Notes List:

Top notes are the first allure to a perfume aroma. They are usually citrus, and eucalyptus oils that gain the most allure to a perfume. Also known as head notes.

- Basil (To Middle)
- Bergamot (To Middle)
- Cajuput
- Cinnamon
- Clary Sage (To Middle)
- Coriander (To Middle)
- Eucalyptus
- Grapefruit
- Hyssop
- Lemon
- Lemongrass (To Middle)
- Lime
- Mandarin
- Neroli (To Middle)
- Niaouli
- Orange
- Peppermint
- Petitgrain

Why Natural Is Best

- Ravensara
- Sage
- Spearmint
- Tagetes
- Tangerine
- Tea Tree (To Middle)
- Thyme (To Middle)
- Verbena

Almost all citrus oils are top notes.

Middle Notes List

The bulk of essential oils are considered middle notes and normally give body to the blend and have a balancing effect. The smells of middle notes are not always immediately evident and may take a couple of minutes to come into their own right and are normally warm and soft fragrances.

Lets look at
The following essential oils are considered

Middle Notes List:-

- Bay
- Black Pepper
- Cardamom
- Chamomile
- Cypress
- Fennel (To Top)
- Geranium
- Ho Leaf
- Ho Wood
- Hyssop
- Juniper
- Lavender (To Top)
- Marjoram
- Melissa (To Top)
- Myrtle
- Nutmeg

- Palma Rosa
- Pine
- Rosemary
- Spikenard
- Yarrow

Base Notes List

Essential oils that are classified as base notes are normally "heavy" oils with their fragrance evident, but will also slowly evolve and be present for a long time and slows down the evaporation of the other oils.

These fragrances are normally intense and heady. They are normally rich and relaxing in nature and are also the most expensive of all oils.

The following essential oils are considered

Base Notes List:

- Balsam Peru
- Champaca
- Cassia (To Middle)
- Cedarwood
- Cinnamon (To Middle)
- Clove
- Frankincense
- Ginger (To Middle)
- Jasmine
- Myrrh
- Oakmoss (Now on the perfumers list of a banned oil.)
- Patchouli
- Rose
- Rosewood (To Middle)
- Sandalwood
- Valerian
- Vanilla
- Vetiver
- Ylang Ylang (To Middle)

Why Natural Is Best

Heavily Aromatic Oils

Blending does not only rely on the notes alone, since some oils are extremely aromatic and, in some cases, overpoweringly so.

When using these very strongly aromatic oils, it is best to add one drop of oil, at a time. This will prevent it from overpowering your entire blend.

Absolutes

I am going to start with my warnings here:-
As I keep an eye on what others are adding to their perfume training course I have observed some of them are either telling you to do what is illegal or unsafe. How they get away with it troubles me.

Porcini mushroom absolute is a very earthy scent to add to wilder type men and womens perfume. However, what you read on the internet and in books can lead you to believe their statement to be true. Trust me this is not an absolute you should use in perfume making, without many years of experience. It is wonderful in chocolate or other dishes but be warned it will send perfume mouldy. Especially as you are a beginner and have probably seen it in perfume recipes/formulas, I am warning you to wit until you decide on natural or synthetic perfumes before you venture down the tack of using rare additives.

Absinthe

Why is absinthe illegal?
Absinthe is regulated by the Food and Drug Administration and, until recently, was completely banned in the U.S. and most of Europe. The reason for this is that absinthe contains thujone, a toxic chemical found in several edible plants including tarragon, sage, and wormwood.

Benzoin

Is added by many perfumers on their website list of ingredients. In my class we will not be using it. We are going to make pure essential oil perfumes, cream perfumes and explore the right way to add alcohol to your blends. Benzoin is a fixative known as a resin and is great for soap making. But not for natural perfumes. Yes it's a natural product

Fixative- Natural

Slows down the rate of evaporation of the most volatile ingredients of a perfume. Cedarwood (Virgina), Cistis, Clarysage, Fir Needle, Frankincense, Helichrysum, Oakmoss, Patchouli, Sandalwood, Sweet Myrrh, Vetiver, Ylang-ylang.

May I Suggest you print this file from this website out and begin your research of essential oils. Click the link or type into the browser

https://en.wikibooks.org/wiki/Complete_Guide_to_Essential_Oils/A_to_Z_of_essential_oils

In description add contra-indications for each oil.

Your Essential Oil List Headings Might Be

Essential oil, Perfumery note , Family, Substitute with, Contra-Indications, Information, Purchased Date, Reorder, Date in,

The family will be the scent family not the botanical name or you can have both listed.

For example, Amyris oil would be under the family of "Fresh-Woody" as it is a bark. It is also a fixative. It could also be a substitute for Sandalwood, although Amyris has a peppery top note within its aroma range.

A Essential oil	B Perfumery note	C Family	D Subsitute with	E Contra-indications	F Information	G Purchased Date	H Reorder	I Date
					Amyris Balsamifera Bark Oil.			
Amyris Bark	Base to mid with a peppery top note	Fresh	For Sandlewood	Non known	Amyris is also known as West Indian Sandalwood or Balsam Torchwood. It does have a beautifully balsamic aroma and is very similar on dry down to Sandalwood oil but has a slightly peppery top note. A fixative			
Angelica	Base							
Anise	Top	Spicy						
Balsam, Peru	Base							
Basil	Top	Herbal						
Bay	Middle							
Bay Laurel	Top							
Benzoin	Base	Resin/ Sweet						

Signature / Perfume Compound Blending

In the signature/perfume compound we need
7. a base note
8. a middle
9. a top note.
10. Plus, a fixative - yet some essential oil automatically work as a fixative.
11. Do not use resins/gums or CO2 oils until you have had more training.

To get the compound right and still call it natural for your sales is a very hard call. This section of the book has troubled me for weeks. How do I condense the information that has taken me many decades to lean into a small "How To Book"?

My end thoughts are I cannot give you years of study all in one book.

I need to keep it as simple as possible - so you can all experience the joy of natural home-made fragrances. Thus, saving you a load of money and adding to the healing powers of being creative and yet still understand the main contra-indications.

DIY Signature Perfume Creating

If people are sensitive to perfumes, they are more than likely going to be sensitive to a natural perfume as well.
There is a big difference between making a perfume for yourself and making them to sell.

If you stick to the blending tables and learn the contra-indications of the oils you choose - you should be safe to go.

Your recommendation in your leaflet should be something like this. :-

All perfumes natural or not can cause reactions in some people. If you are sensitive to perfumes, we suggest you do as our ancestors did and wear the perfume on your petticoat, a handkerchief tucked into your bra, (brassiere}, a timber medallion or on cotton wool ball in a locket.

Next add any contra -indications for the oils you have used such as

Example

Warning this fragrance is not suitable if you are Pregnant or Lactating (breastfeeding)
This warning would go into your leaflet inside the box.
On the outside of box state: -
"Warning not suitable while pregnant".

I the author Robyn have used - being pregnant as an example for you the reader/student, because in my test compound I have added oils pregnant womenfolk cannot use plus the mix of essential oil compound mix, ratio to base oil is too high.

Oils not to use in pregnancy at all:
Basil, Cedarwood, Fennel, Clary Sage, Myrrh, Marjoram, Sage, Peppermint, Thyme.

Why Natural Is Best

To Increase Lactation:
Anise, Fennel, Lemongrass, Jasmine

To Decrease Lactation:
Mint, Parsley, Sage.
Lets say you have added Fennel to the signature/perfume compound then you would add a warning

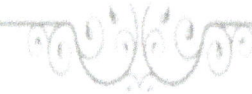

Don't sweat the small stuff.

Just create first for yourself.
1. Make several Signature/perfume compounds
2. Document ever drop you place in each test bottle.
3. Then when you have created the aroma you love
4. Allow to sit for six weeks or more so all oil aromas mellow or merge together.
5. Mix it with your base oil or cream. (for a more natural perfume or with alcohol for a standard unnatural perfume.
6. Hygiene- Be sure to filter your perfume and use only clean containers to store them in. You don't want to introduce bacteria, fungi, or mould into your perfume, nor do you want to encourage their growth. Many essential oils inhibit microbial growth, so this is less of an issue with perfume, however, it can become more of a concern if you dilute the perfume to make cologne.
7. Then look up the contra- indications of the essential oils you have added to your chosen test signature If there is an oil added then you do not wear it on your skin. You wear it on a timber necklace or in a locket or other methods I have suggested above. And in the section heading named "**Marketing**"

Signature Perfume

Test Mixing

It is important that you now read from here down to about page 120. Then get some coloured water, bottles, talc and some cream, and pretend you are doing what I am explaining. Because just reading as you go will not make complete sense. Or actually get all your kit out and go through the steps, as you read.

I love to start my compounds in a clear glass jug, beaker, or bottle, because watching the perfume compound being make excites me. It is a cheap thrill but, hey, who cares every dash of happiness in life should be embraced with great delight.

I also start mixing when the sun catches my crystals hanging in my window. The rainbows in many places on my walls from the crystals also adds a marvelous uplift to my mood. My dog is always very excited when I wake up in the morning and loves his cuddle and a kiss. Because he is excited that I am awake - he also lifts my mood.

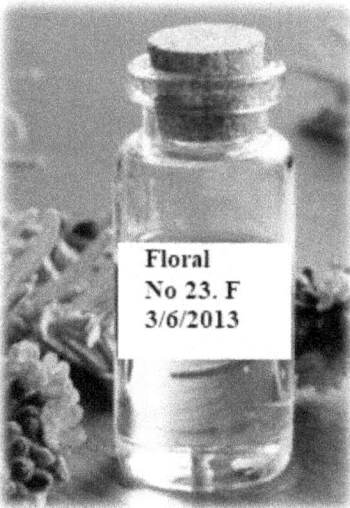

Floral
No 23. F
3/6/2013

Why Natural Is Best

In the morning when you wake up, you need to decide how you feel.

Be organized and at one with yourself.

Never start before you have had your cuppa, made your bed, been for an early morning walk and balanced your chakras. You're showered and dressed for success, chores are done, tick.

Be in the most malleolusly alive - state of mind.

5. Organize a beautiful work space with everything you need.
6. Turn your phone onto silent.
7. Decide on which "Note Family" you are going to create. As a sample I am going to walk you through a Romantic Floral Note.

Example Of A Signature Compound.

Use three to eight essential oils
Put them in your test bottle or glass beaker one drop at time and smell as you go.
I am using 4 fragrances

12. Start with the base notes put maybe 3 drops
13. Build with one drop of each of the other notes
14. Next the middle notes
15. Next the top note
16. Shake, keep building one drop at a time, small and decide.
17. Last add the essential oil you have chosen as your fixative. Add it one drop at a time.
18. Six week or more rest time is needed
19. Then you add it to your chosen base be that a carrier oil, a cream, talc or alcohol.
20. You will do this in about 3 or more test bottles, adding different amounts of each note. To each test and write down what you are adding to each test bottle.

By Robyn Ji Smith   page. 108

DIY Signature Perfume Creating

Here are tests I did

Base notes I had on my table were
Frankincense, Ylang Ylang, Patchouli, Vetiver

Middle Notes
Basil, Rose Geranium, Melissa

Top Notes
Eucalyptus, Bergamot, Orange, Lavender, Lime

Lavender is classed as a top note but does the work of a base note and a fixative

My test bottles were narrow neck 50 ml Blue glass. With a eyedropper lid. For six weeks after making these signature perfume compounds, I kept in my pantry on the bottom shelve.

Signature tests 1 & 2

Test One		Test two
5 drops of Frankincense	base	3 drops Frankincense
5 drops of Patchouli	base	10 drops Patchouli
6 drops of Melissa	middle	5 drops Vetiver
10 drops Rose geranium	middle	15 drops of Rose geranium
3 drops Eucalyptus	top	1 drops Eucalyptus
4 drops Bergamot	top	7 drops Bergamot
3 drops of lime	top	1 drops of lime
5 drops Lavender	Middle Fixative	3 drops lavender

This is a perfume compound and must not be put onto the skin. You must now blend it with base oil

Why Natural Is Best

1. I put the base notes in each test bottle first. Adding different quantities to each test bottle. Although I have the total written here for each oil they did not go in in this quantity, at once.
2. Next the middle notes
3. Then the top notes
4. To tie it all together I added lavender to both tests, *I also find Frankincense and Myrrh are good fixatives.*
5. Due to frankincense being a wax you could heat slightly now and run through a coffee filter or wait for the aromas to blend *(6 weeks)* then heat gently. Sometimes the essential oil of Frankincense is already melted in an essential oil form.

6. However, it will often reset in the bottle and go dark. It is a tricky oil as it is actually a wax so buy from a supplier who loves their trade. You can also buy it in liquid form 3% in Jojoba base oil.

7. I waited six weeks for the aroma to musically blend. Then heated gently and gave it a good shake.

8. Put through coffee filter.
9. Then added to a base oil and a cocoa butter. base.

You need to be experimental.

The base can be: -
   A. Talc,
   B. Creams,
   C. Cold Pressed oils *as per the list of base oils.*

Oil Burners & Diffusers

It is best to only put one to three essential oils in a diffuser. When I was at college studying oils our class was told by the scientist - that electric pulse type diffusers send essential oils aroma molecules toxic. To only defuse or vaporize in a double glazed or triple glazed oil burner or a glass one. Oil burners when single glazed can get hot and explode.

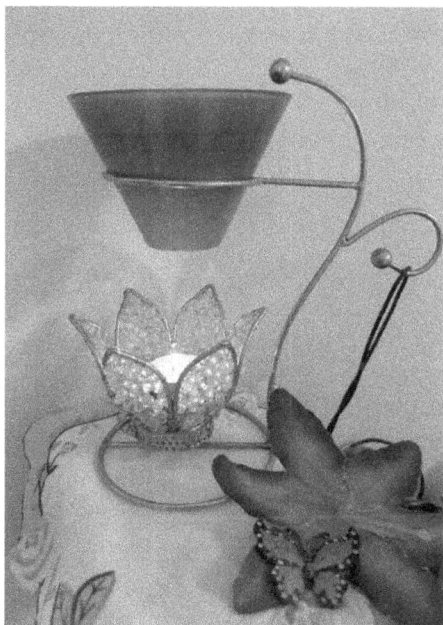

Candles come in 2 to 9 hours burn time. I buy the four-hour candles as that is the amount of time you should vaporize essential oils for. Longer and your olfactory sensors become over loaded and the cilia stops dancing.

If you are going to make compounds to sell as diffusing oils only use 2-3 oils and be sure they are safe to diffuse. Sell in small bottles or they will be too expensive for the average house holder to buy.

You can make different aromas or healing compounds but you need to be careful not to give them healing names.

Be Marvelously Alive.

Why Natural Is Best

Here are a few ideas:-

Oil Burner Aromas.

- Floral
- Air Refresher
- Winter Lift
- Home Refresher
- Dinner Party Mood Lifter
- Gog Odour Evaporator.

Humidity is important in your home
I put lemon grass plants in a saucepan of water and one drop
of essential oil of lemongrass.

Chromatography

Definition of chromatography. : a process in which a chemical
mixture carried by a liquid or gas is separated into
components as a result of differential distribution of the
solutes as they flow around or over a stationary liquid or solid
phase.

Honey producing bees and humans have their own built in
chromatography. With humans it works mainly through the
olfactory system, eg aromas.

I liked this video.
https://www.youtube.com/watch?v=I1YppupsNOU

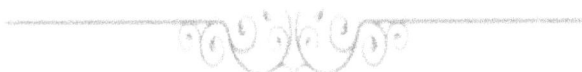

Natural Perfume Mix

A perfume compound is all essential oils a perfume mix is when you put a small quantity of the compound aroma into a base.

Natural 1

In a 50ml Blue narrow neck bottle with an eye dropper as a lid.
I added 49ml of Sweet Apricot oil
12 drops of Compound test one

Natural Perfume 2

In a 50ml Blue narrow neck bottle with an eye dropper as a lid.
I added 49ml of Olive oil
15 drops of Compound test Two

Perfume 3 and 3a

In two 10ml roll on bottles
I added 9ml Alcohol
5 drops of compound test one in one bottle and
6 drops of compound test two in the other bottle

Perfume 4 and 4a

In two 10ml roll on bottles
I added 9ml Olive oil
5 drops of Natural Perfume Mix 3a in one bottle and
6 drops of Natural Perfume 3 in the other bottle

Talc – Kaolin

I use and like corn starch and talc mixed together as I use it as a deodorant.

3/4 cup Arrowroot powder Or Talc or corn-starch
1/4 cup Kaolin Clay.
1 tbsp. Magnesium Carbonate powder or Baking Soda
10 drops Lavender essential oil (optional)

Be Marvelously Alive.   **113** | P a g e

Why Natural Is Best

5 drops Ylang Ylang essential oil (optional)
5 drops Rose essential oil (optional)

Choose whatever oils you like or add your compound perfume

Talc Test 1
I added 15 drop of test 1 to one tablespoon of base oil of
Jojoba,
Stirred well into 200 grams of Talc

Talc Test 2
And 15 drops of test 2 compound to three tablespoons of
jojoba oil in another 200 grams of talc, in a separate jar.
Shake well. Put the lid on.
I allow these to sit for a few days then put each mixture into a
blender and back into the jar.

Vaporizers

In two 30 ml Blue glass bottles with dripolators
I added 50 drops of each compound to each bottle and toped
up with apricot oil.

However, a two or three oil blend is better for vaporizing.

Your warning leaflet should state.

Photosensitive do not wear on skin if going into the sun
for longer than an hour as there are citrus oils added.
Unsuitable for women while pregnant or breast feeding.
Use a perfume pendant.
or
Frankincense added. Warning to women that are pregnant
or best feeding.
Do not use this fragrance while pregnant or brest feeding.
or
Due to the fresh aromas of citrus it is advised that this
perfume could be photosensitive in some individuals.
Or

Warning Photosensitive in some individuals. If pregnant or nursing do not apply to skin
Or
Application to the skin may increase sensitivity to sunlight. Not suitable for pregnant or nursing mothers.

Signature Perfume Blending

Have your entire perfume kit set out ready to use.
Your signature /perfume compounds test are setting in front of
you or at least the one you have decided you feel uplifted by
and now want to make a natural perfume.

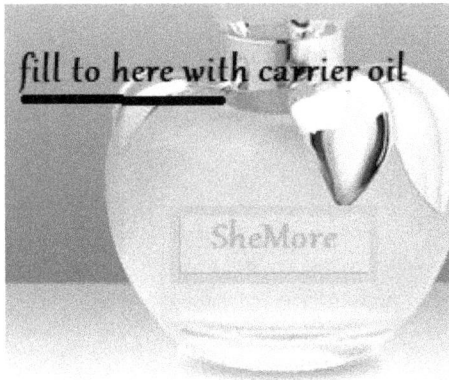

Signature Perfume Blend 5
In 50ml bottle with an eyedropper I placed
12 drops of test one compound
48 ml fractionated coconut oil
Placed bottle in saucepan and gently heated to blend the
frankincense.

Signature Perfume Blend 6
In 50ml bottle with an eyedropper I placed
20 drops of test one compound
47 ml cold pressed apricot oil.
Placed bottle in saucepan and gently heated to blend the
frankincense.

Signature Perfume Blend 7

A small glass jar
12 drops of test one compound
Filled the jar with shea butter.
I gently heated the butter and the perfume compound together before placing in the jar.
As the glass was a clear glass jar I pasted gift paper on the jar to prevent light from entering the jar.

Signature Perfume Blend 8

1. A small glass jar
2. 20 drops of test one compound
3. Filled the jar with Talc.
4. I gently heated the perfume compound in a separate jar in a pan of hot water my setting on the stove was low.
5. I used a glass stirring stick and mixed the warm compound into 10ml of olive oil.
6. Then added to the talc.
7. I then put the mixture through a cake sieve, onto baking paper and put into a jar.
8. As the glass was a clear glass jar I pasted gift paper on the jar to prevent light from entering the jar.
9. I then added a powder puff to the jar.
10. Test signatures 5 to 8 were exactly the same as the above 4 tests but I replaced test one compound with **test two compound**.

Decorating jars can be a load of fun and very therapeutic. Here is one YouTube site but there are plenty of other tutorials
https://youtu.be/Zx6PRLCGWUI

For massage blends I add my signature/perfume compounds straight into a small bottle of base oil usually olive oil.

Why Natural Is Best

> I dip the lid in hot wax that I melt in an empty tuna tin in a pan of water.

> Then I place baby photos of the person I am giving the oil to as a gift onto the bottle with PVA glue. I also love to use wrapping paper or old newspapers.

Eau-de-cologne compound

We are going to examine "Eau-de-cologne compound"

What is the difference between perfume and eau de cologne?

The difference is simply the amount or concentration of oils in the fragrance.

Eau de parfum has a higher concentration than eau de toilette, making it a stronger fragrance.

There is also pure perfume, which has the highest concentration, and eau de cologne, which has the lowest concentration of oils.

First A Natural Eau-de-cologne compound

In a 100ml Blue glass bottle add
10 Drops Bergamot
5 Drops Neroli
4 Drops Lemon
2 Drops Orange
Add 98ml Jojoba oil

Second Not so natural Eau-de-cologne compound
In a 100ml Blue glass bottle add
10 Drops Bergamot
5 Drops Neroli
4 Drops Lemon
2 Drops Orange
Add 10ml Jojoba oil

By Robyn Ji Smith   page. 118

DIY Signature Perfume Creating

Half ill bottle with alcohol.
Put lid on and shake well
Fill bottle now with spring water.

Keeping A Diary And Inventory.

For many reasons when making a perfume it is important to document what you have put into the bottle.

DIY perfumers will probably keep the recipe in a perfume diary just like a recipe book.

If you are going to make and sell perfumes then far more information is required. You need to become a geek/ nerd.

Why Study Essential Oil

This is a brief explanation on where study might begin.

To study oils takes many years and under guidance.

However, for a DIY perfumer a full study is not necessary as long as you know the contra-indications and the blending factors which I have out lined above.

My main point here is for you to understand you need to stick to the above methods and do not sway because essential oils are every bit as complicated as the human mind and body.

You can access the power of essential oils many ways, but the most common practices include aromatic diffusion, topical application, and dietary consumption. These methods bring the pure essence of health-promoting botanicals to your home, family, and life.

Why Natural Is Best

Note *consumption can only be allowed if directed by a Certified Aromatherapist and with the therapist grade oils diluted perfectly for each individual. The law otherwise is "Nil By Mouth".*

Essential Oils If you have ever enjoyed the scent of a rose, you've experienced the aromatic qualities of essential oils. These naturally occurring, volatile aromatic compounds are found in the seeds, bark, stems, roots, flowers, and other parts of plants. They can be both beautifully and powerfully fragrant. Essential oils give plants their distinctive smells, essential oils protect plants and play a role in plant pollination. In addition to their intrinsic benefits to plants and their beautiful fragrance.

Essential oils have enhanced lives for thousands of years, offering a variety of benefits from cosmetic and dietary purposes to spiritual and religious use. Extracted through careful steam distillation, resin tapping, and cold pressing, the purest essential oils are far more powerful than the botanicals from which they come.

The term "essential oil" is a contraction of the original "quintessential oil."

This stems from the Aristotelian idea that matter is composed of four elements, namely-

- Fire,
- Air,
- Earth,
- Water.
- Life Force

The fifth element, or quintessence, was then considered to be spirit or life force. Distillation and evaporation were thought to be processes of removing the spirit from the plant and this is also reflected in our language since the term "spirits" is used to describe distilled alcoholic beverages such as brandy, whiskey, and eau de vie. The last of these again shows reference to the concept of removing the life force from the plant. Nowadays, of course, we know that, far from being spirit, essential oils are physical in nature and composed of complex mixtures of chemicals.

The International Organization for Standardization (ISO) in their Vocabulary of Natural Materials (ISO/D1S9235.2) defines an essential oil as a product made by distillation

with either water or steam or by mechanical processing of citrus rinds or by dry distillation of natural materials. Following the distillation, the essential oil is physically separated from the water phase.

EO Chemistry Outline

Chemistry is not all that important to make a simple DIY perfume if you follow some basic blending rules, which I have added to this book for the simplicity of DIY perfumes.

However, if you are going to make perfumes with alcohol or just make pure blends to sell at markets the more you know the better.

What Exactly Functional Groups Are, And What They Have To Do With The Chemistry Of Essential Oils?

In a nutshell: functional groups are small groups of atoms within molecules. They importantly contribute to their physical properties,

- such as solubility,

- melting and boiling points,

As well as determine their chemical reactivity – kinds of chemical reactions they may undergo in various conditions.

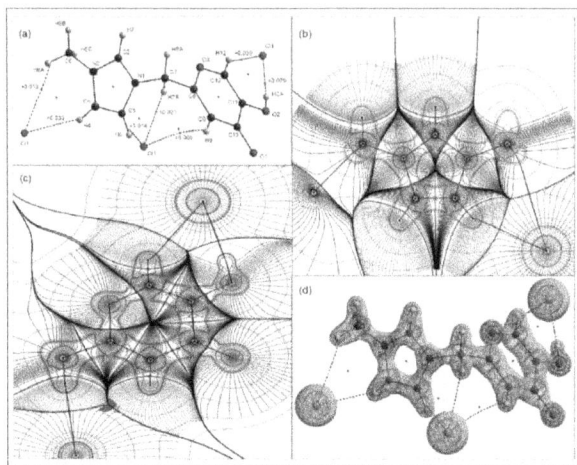

For further reading click here.

https://www.researchgate.net/figure/Results-of-quantum-theory-of-atoms-in-molecules-applied-for-MIKCl-a-Critical_fig11_284407453

Organic chemistry is essentially the chemistry of compounds that contain carbon and hydrogen atoms.

Other elements bring new properties to organic compounds, oxygen being by far the most important in essential oils. Depending on how oxygen combines with carbon and hydrogen atoms, different types of molecules may form:

- alcohols,

- aldehydes,

- ketones,

- acids,

- esters,

DIY Signature Perfume Creating

- ethers,

- oxides

- lactones –

each characterized by the specific functional group.

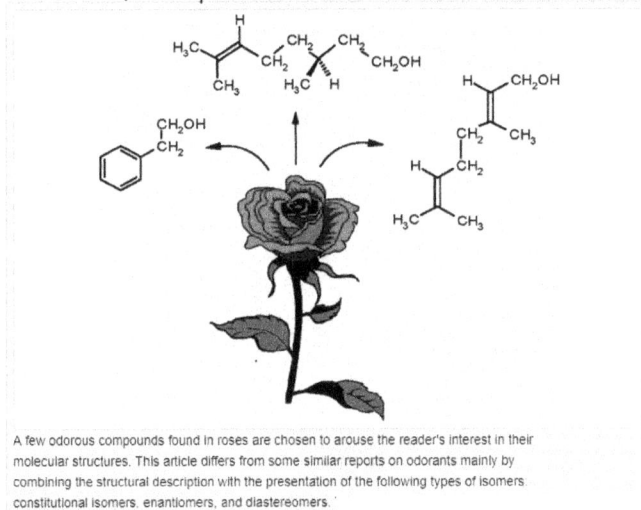

Abstract ~ *Odoriferous Compounds in Rose Damask Essential Oil*

A few odorous compounds found in roses are chosen to arouse the reader's interest in their molecular structures. This article differs from some similar reports on odorants mainly by combining the structural description with the presentation of the following types of isomers: constitutional isomers, enantiomers, and diastereomers.

Rose Otto has over 500 different healing chemical components.

Rose Otto Essential Oil is lighter in color and thinner in viscosity than Rose CO2 Extract or Rose Absolute. However, Rose Otto Essential Oil is more costly than the absolute because it takes significantly more rose petals to produce Rose Otto than it does to product the absolute.

Rose water has the same fragrance and is very inexpensive by comparison., but will not have the same strength chemical healing properties as the essential oil. But great for perfumers.

I like the info about rose oil on this site

https://www.aromaweb.com/essential-oils/rose-oil.asp

Essential Oils Functional Groups

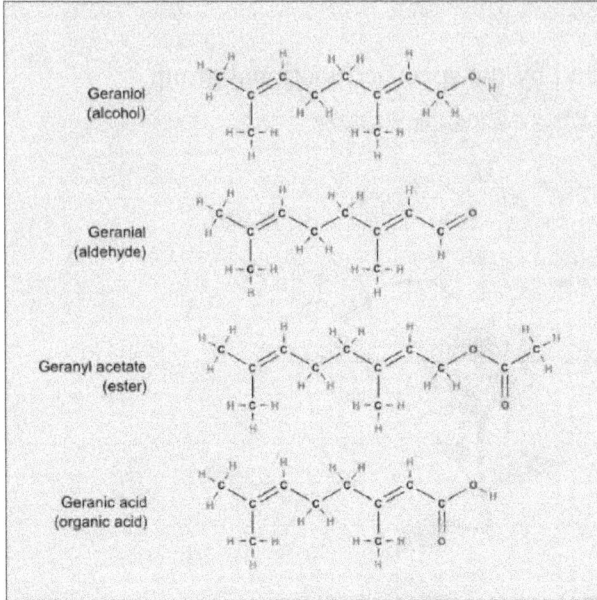

Different functional groups on the same molecular backbone
(geranyl– in this case). The position and bonding of oxygen
(O) to carbon (C) and hydrogen (H) gives rise to different
types of molecules

(note that geranic acid is not typically a constituent of
essential oils, however, it is sometimes found in the
hydrolats).

Knowing your oils' composition according to chemical
families can help you predict certain physical properties, or
how long they will keep and whether you should store them in
a refrigerator. To some degree, you may also infer on the
distribution and metabolism of the constituents in the body.

However, with the recent essential oil chemistry hype, it may
seem to a newcomer that you can't even smell an oil without

knowing how to draw a cyclic monoterpene. It's important to understand that classification of compounds according to their chemical structure is not something new or exclusive to aromatherapy. It's the basis for studying the biochemistry of plant volatiles: how they continuously transform from one to another in different parts of cells and plant organs, like in a giant recycling assembly system, and how various factors influence these transformations.

Chemistry also concerns changes of essential oils during and after distillation, as well as analytics. But as soon as individual constituents enter the body, we rather talk about their pharmacokinetics and pharmacodynamics.

Pierre Franchomme, a French naturopath, conducted a series of experiments in the 1980's. In co-operation with Jean Mars, he devised a measuring system where he dispersed aerosols (tiny droplets) of isolated essential oil constituents on a charged electrode. By measuring changes in electric current, he deduced their degree of ionisation, the ability to gain or lose electric charge (Franchomme and Pénoël 1990/2001).

Depending on the direction of electric current obtained, the compounds were assigned as either positive (electron accepting) or negative (electron donating). The positioning of compounds with same functional groups to a confined area on a two-dimensional diagram, where the vertical axis represents the degree and direction of ionisation, and the horizontal axis represents the degree of polarity, was for the authors a proof that they have similar properties.

Why Natural Is Best

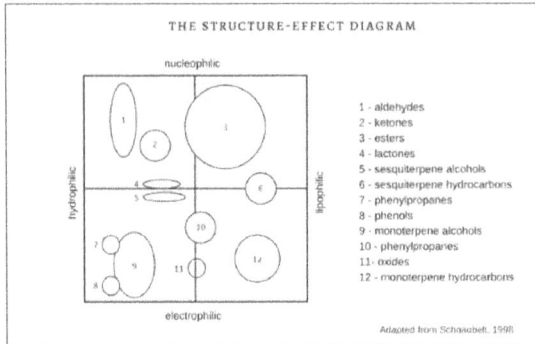

THE STRUCTURE-EFFECT DIAGRAM

1 - aldehydes
2 - ketones
3 - esters
4 - lactones
5 - sesquiterpene alcohols
6 - sesquiterpene hydrocarbons
7 - phenylpropanes
8 - phenols
9 - monoterpene alcohols
10 - phenylpropanes
11- oxides
12 - monoterpene hydrocarbons

Adapted from Schnaubelt, 1998

Diagram and method explained in

Advanced Aromatherapy (1998) by Dr Kurt Schnaubelt.

A more simple quick to the point, explanation about chemistry that will suit DIY perfumers can be found **In "Foolproof Aromatherapy "By** Robyna Smith -Keys

Extracting Oils From Flowers And Herbs.

DIY Enfleurage

Enfleurage Is typically used for delicate flowers such as Jasmin, Lilacs and other tiny petal flowers.

Jasmin grow quickly in large pots or garden beds. You do need a very large amount of these tiny petals and you must pick them early in the morning while the dew is still on the petals.

Enfleurage is a very old technique of extracting the aromatic oils from flowers that was popularized in France during the 19th century. It works on the simple principle that fats dissolve essential oils and thereby absorb

their aromas. ... The oil saturated fat, called a pomade, was then dissolved by alcohol.

Process

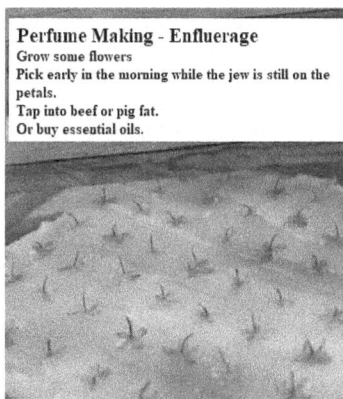

Perfume Making - Enfluerage
Grow some flowers
Pick early in the morning while the jew is still on the petals.
Tap into beef or pig fat.
Or buy essential oils.

There are two types of processes:

Cold Enfleurage

In cold enfleurage, a large framed plate of glass, called a chassis, is smeared with a layer of animal fat, usually lard or tallow (from pork or beef, respectively), and allowed to set. Botanical matter, usually petals or whole flowers, is then placed on the fat and its scent is allowed to diffuse into the fat over the course of 1–3 days. The process is then repeated by replacing the spent botanicals with fresh ones until the fat has reached a desired degree of fragrance saturation.

This procedure was developed in southern France

in the 18th century for the production of high-grade concentrates.

Hot Enfleurage

This is better and quicker it is also less trouble as the fat does not have time to go off. In hot enfleurage, solid fats are heated and botanical matter is stirred into the fat. Spent botanicals are repeatedly strained from the fat and replaced with fresh material until the fat is saturated with fragrance. This method is considered the oldest known procedure for preserving plant fragrance substances.

In both instances, once the fat is saturated with fragrance, it is then called the "enfleurage pomade". The enfleurage pomade was either sold as it was, or it could be further washed or soaked in ethyl alcohol to draw the fragrant molecules into the alcohol. The alcohol was then separated from the fat and allowed to evaporate, leaving behind the absolute of the botanical matter. The spent fat is usually used to make soaps since it is still relatively fragrant.

The enfleurage fragrance extraction method is one of the oldest. It is also highly inefficient and costly but was the sole method of extracting the fragrant compounds in delicate flowers such as jasmine and tuberose, which would be destroyed or denatured by the high temperatures required by methods of fragrance extraction such as steam distillation.

The method is now superseded by more efficient techniques such as solvent extraction or supercritical fluid extraction using supercritical carbon dioxide (CO_2) or similar compressed gases.

But this antient method can be done at home. I prefer to use coconut oil because the pork or beef fat attracts flies and develops a very unpleasant odour.

Tinctures & Infusions

Many Youtubers say to place them in a zip lock bag. **Do not do this, plastic is a very toxic medium.**

1. Wash your petals or herbs

2. Or pick in the early morn while it is raining

3. Pat dry gently with a towel

4. Place your petals in a glass jar

5. Add A base oil like Olive, jojoba or almond oil

6. Stir in a stabbing method to puncture the flower petals or herbs with a timber spoon

7. Place cooking paper on the jar under the lid

8. Allow to sit for about a week.

9. Shake the jar every day during that week.

10. Strain through gauge cloth into a clean jar.

11. Repeat steps 1-9 several times. Adding more petals every few days if you have enough in your garden. But do not add more base oil step 5.

When you are happy with the aroma after straining through the gauze fabric you have your aromatic oil.

You can also use alcohol as a base in place of oil. The aromatic/fragrant oil and the alcohol will merge. Therefore, it is important to repeat steps 1 – 9 many times.

Do not use vegetable oils from a supermarket they have bleach in them and they can cause allergic reactions in most humans. However most olive oils are cold pressed and can be purchased at a supermarket but read the label and be sure it is pure.

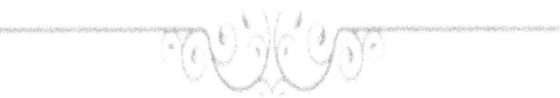

Steam Distilling

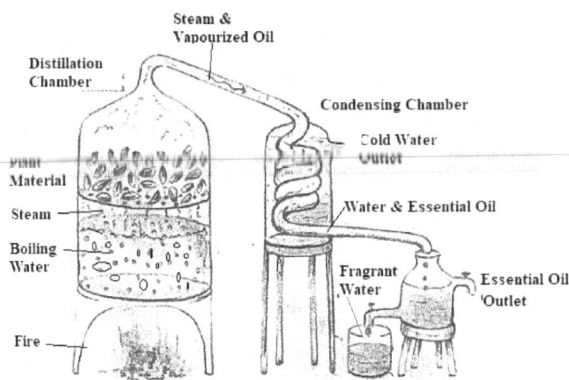

If you start with the fire and follow the above diagram up and over to the right you will get the message.

Cold Pressing Oils

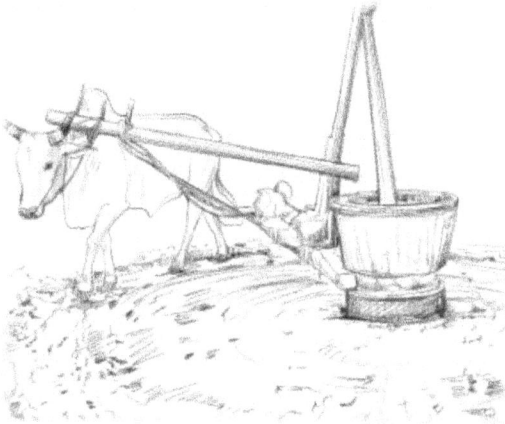

By far the purest method of extracting essential oils and base carrier oils. Cold pressing is always used before but also prior to hot pressing.

Expression (Cold Pressing)

Expression or cold pressing is commonly used in the production of essential and food oils. The term expression refers to any physical process in which the essential oil glands in the biomass are crushed or broken to release the oil. The resulting oil–water emulsion is typically separated by centrifugation. Traditionally, cold pressing was conducted by hand; however, for large-scale commercialization, this is impractical. Thus, with the advancement of industrialization, a number of machines have been designed to achieve the same results on commercial scale.

It is important to note that oils extracted using this method have a relatively short shelf life.

Therefore, when choosing essential oils for your natural blend you need to know by which method it was distilled. Your shelf life will be shorter when using a mixture of essential oils. This is important to note that a natural perfume should only be added to small bottles and jars.

The Olfactory System -Smell

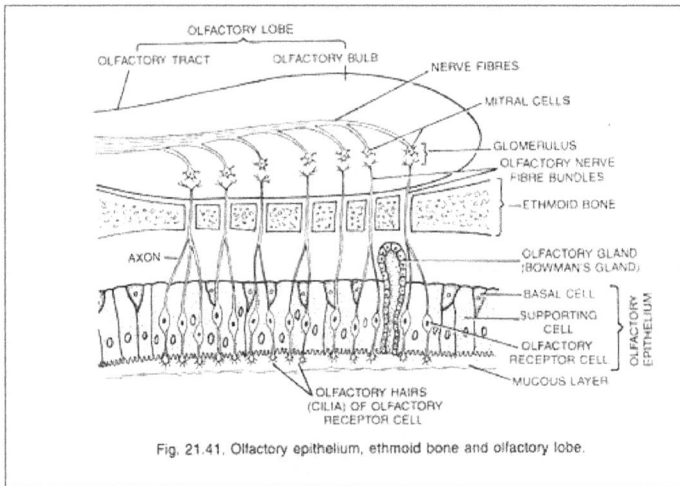

Fig. 21.41, Olfactory epithelium, ethmoid bone and olfactory lobe.

In the base of this diagram you will see the cilia they are hairs that dance constantly and they are the receptors you need to enchant when making perfumes. If you do not like the smell it will actually make you sick.

Olfaction is a chemoreception that, through the sensory olfactory system, forms the perception of smell.

Olfaction has many purposes, such as the detection of hazards, pheromones, and food.

Olfaction occurs when odorants bind to specific sites on olfactory receptors located in the nasal cavity.

Glomeruli aggregate signals from these receptors and transmit them to the olfactory bulb, where the sensory input will start to interact with parts of the brain responsible for smell identification, memory, and emotion.

Olfactory dysfunction arises as the result of many different peripheral and central disturbances, including upper respiratory infections, traumatic brain injury, and neurodegenerative disease.

Smells can do may things to people.

They can lift their mood or cause them to dislike the smell and hate your product. Test your compound aromas on people outside your personal friend group to get a better gauge of how they will please or be dismissed.

Essential Oils-Comparing prices and substitutes

Above I gave you a list of oils that can be substituted with other oils. One reason might be you do not have the oil you need to use on that day. Another reason might be the price, or the healing chemicals. At this point if you are a DIY perfumer starting this fascinating journey it is probably the price.

Let us look at the worlds most adorable two fragrances Sandalwood and Rose Otto

Substituting Sandalwood with Amyris
They certainly differ in price. One reason might be that a sandalwood tree needs to be grown and cared for - for 25 years or more before the timber is perfumed to the right components/chemicals before - it becomes aromatic enough for both healing purposes and perfume making.

Why Natural Is Best

Sandalwood is relatively rare and is the second most expensive wood in the world (after African blackwood). It retains its unique fragrance for decades. It's expensive and rare because it is slow-growing and in recent decades has been over-harvested due to high commercial demand, especially in India.

Where a plant is grown will also be of importance in healing properties. This is due to Photosynthesis the process by which green plants and some other organisms use sunlight to synthesize nutrients from carbon dioxide and water. Photosynthesis in plants generally involves the green pigment chlorophyll and generates oxygen as a by-product.

Because sandalwood is relatively rare and is the second most expensive wood in the world (after African blackwood). It retains its unique fragrance for decades. It's expensive and rare because it is slow-growing and in recent decades has been over-harvested due to high commercial demand, especially in India.

Amyris oil and sandal oil predominantly differ in their chemical composition, resulting in different smell, but above all, different therapeutic properties. Sandal oils contain a high amount of santalol and its derivatives (nearly 70% in Santalum album; up to 35% in Santalum spicatum). These compounds are not present in Amyris oil, which mainly contains beta-caryophyllen (up to 20%), d-cadinene, amyroline, etc. On the other hand, these compounds are not found in sandal oil.

Amyris trees once upon a time took 30 years of growth before the wood was mature enough to make amyris oil. But now they are grown on large plantations in order to make furniture.

At the same time, it allows to produce cheap amyris oil from twigs, tree branches and industrial production waste. It is worth pointing out that such oil may have irritating and allergenic properties. Naming it "West Indian Sandalwood Oil" facilitate only its sale to unaware clients. Contrary to Amyris oil, sandal oil of Indian origin is expensive due to economic reasons. Sandal trees are rare and difficult to grow; therefore, the oil is mainly produced from industrial waste (production of furniture or trinkets). Australian sandalwood oil obtained from Santalum spicata is less expensive, but due to chemical composition, its therapeutic properties are not as valuable as Santalum Album Oil.

Just like Lavender grown on the mainland of Australia is not as therapeutic as Lavender grown in Tasmania.

The long and the short storey here is:
You are buying essential oils for perfume making so if you can source a cheaper version of the aroma you are in creation of. You are now forewarned or enlightened. But if you look around you can get Sandalwood for much the same price.

The comparisons here are Amyris 8ml is $149
Sandalwood for 17ml is $187 and double the quantity. Therefore, 17ml gives you over 1700 drops of oil and as a blend may only need a few drops ask the supplier if you can just buy 5 ml. Sandalwood also has 10 years shelf-life and is a fixative that will hold all your aromas together.

17 ml Sandalwood Australian Certified Organic Oil
Product number: OC17SANDAUST

AU$187.00

1

Why Natural Is Best

Australian Sandalwood
Pure Essential Oil 8ml

$149.95

IN ESSENCE®

Australian
Sandalwood

Pure Essential Oil

IN ESSENCE®
Australian
Sandalwood

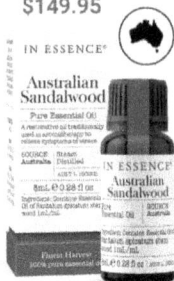

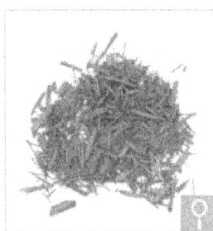

17 ml Amyris Wood Essential Oil

Product number: OE17AMYRISWOOD

AUS$31.90

1

However, my usual suppliers has uncertified Amyris oil 17 ml for just $31.90. This is fine for making perfume.

I have spoken above about Rose oil in my substitution section.

The only way to get a rose sent is with Rose water and rose geranium added to rose oil. Further to this statement you cannot add essential oils to water, they will not blend.

Rose oil is pure and there is no getting its aroma any other way, other than growing a very large amount of roses and distilling the oil yourself. But you can naturally produce a similar aroma.

Let us say we want a rose perfume all natural. To a base oil you could add a few drops of Rose Otto and then add triple that amount of Rose Geranium. You can still call it a rose perfume, after you have added this compound of Rose and Rose Geranium to a base oil or alcohol. Once the alcohol is added you can then safely add some water, or rose water.

Shelf Life

Base oil perfumes will have a two-year self-life. However, that depends on how quickly you use your base ingredients after buying and how quickly you sell them in your end product.

Alcohol perfumes will have about a five-year shelf-life.

How Long Do Essential Oils Last?
For example, in a 2005 study, researchers found that the constituents of sweet fennel oil had completely altered from oxidation when placed under a light for two months. Another study involving Sweet Orange essential oil demonstrated that the oil underwent extreme changes after 50 minutes of exposure to UV light. In fact, 12 new chemical constituents were found in the oil after UV exposure.

There's also some evidence that exposure to high heat can change the chemical balance and makeup of essential oils. While more research is needed to fully grasp the impact that heat has on the essential oils, most manufacturers typically recommend keeping them away from high temperatures or sunlight.

How do you know if your essential oils have surpassed their shelf life? Some, particularly limonene-containing citrus oils like lemon and grapefruit, will have an unpleasant scent. But with most oils, the aroma of oxidation can be less noticeable.

There are other ways to examine whether oxygen has shortened the shelf life of your essential oil. Others, like peppermint and chamomile, will change color; still others may have a noticeable change in their viscosity, (the state of being thick, sticky, and semi-fluid in consistency,)

In all of these cases, the therapeutic benefits of the essential oils when they're applied to your skin or put into a diffuser are degraded or lost. After that deterioration, the products are only beneficial for some skincare applications.

Oils like tea tree and lavender, however, can actually irritate mucous membranes or the skin, or cause sensitization, if used after they've oxidized.

The answer is different for different oils, because they all have different chemical compositions. Most will last at least two years before starting to degrade, unless they contain one of the unstable carrier oils mentioned earlier. And some can last for as long as 15 years without losing their effectiveness.

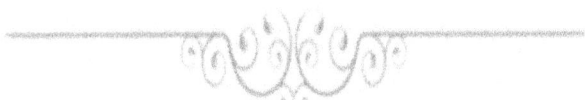

Oils that improve with age.

Many experts advise replacing essential oils every three years to be safe. The exceptions are:

1. Patchouli,

2. Ylang Ylang,

3. Vetiver

4. Sandalwood

These four essential oils actually improve as they age. This is why they are excellent perfume creating oils as they will also improve the shelf-life of other oils.

Here's a categorized list of the essential oil shelf life you can expect, as long as they're treated and stored properly. This will not be clear to the DIY perfumer yet will serve you well should you continue with your chemical study of essential oils.

Why Natural Is Best

As a DIY perfumer - it is a must, that you date the oil the day you purchased the oil. Use good sense and keep away from light, in a cupboard and throw oils out after use by date. Check the list below.

Essential Oil Shelf Life		
Monoterpenes 2 -5 Years	Aldehydes 5 Years	Esters 6 Years
Oxides 4 Years	Ketones 6 Years	Sesquiterpenes 7 -10 Years
Phenols 5 Years	Monoterpinols 6 Years	Sesquiterpenols 6 -10 Years

Sesquiterpene molecules deliver oxygen molecules to cells, like hemoglobin does in the blood.

Sesquiterpenes can also erase or deprogram miswritten codes in **the** DNA. Therefore. you should always consider to have an oil rich in sesquiterpene in your home and use them in oils you are going to blend for healing purposes.

They also have a six to ten-year self-life and are great to have in perfumes as a stabilizer.

Oils containing Sesquiterpenes include:

Cedarwood, Sandalwood and Myrrh have the highest amount of Sesquiterpenes about 70%

Patchouli4,5 bulnesene, guaiene Approximately 65%

Vetiver5 vatirenene, seychellane, cubebene Approximately 65%

DIY Signature Perfume Creating

Carophyllene- found in Lavender, Clary Sage, Marjoram. about 59%

Azulene & Chamazulene- found in Chamomile.
Cadinene- in Patchouli, Lemon, Cedarwood.
Black Pepper caryophyllene Approximately 25%

Ginger zingiberene, sesquiphellandrene, curcumene Approximately 55%

Helichrysum himachalene, curcumene Approximately 40%

Myrrh sesquiterpenoid, elemene Approximately 55%

Ylang Ylang germacrene, caryophyllene, farnesene Approximately 55%

Stability Testing

Let us look to the future.
If you want to become very professional you need very good documentation.

Every time you place a new order for an essential oil or raw products you need the safety data sheet in your files.

This is a typical eucalyptus safety sheet I received with my eucalyptus oil. I have only take a group photo of this report you can get your own for study purposes **but must be a registered business to receive these.**

Why Natural Is Best

NEW DIRECTIONS LABORATORY

SAFETY DATA SHEET

Page 1 of 13

| Eucalyptus Citriodora Essential Oil – Certified Organic | Issue/Revision Date: | 6th September 2019 |

SECTION 1 – IDENTIFICATION OF THE MATERIAL AND SUPPLIER

1.1 Product Name:	Eucalyptus Citriodora Essential Oil – Certified Organic
1.2 Botanical Name:	Eucalyptus citriodora
1.3 Product Code:	OCEUCACITR
1.4 Synonyms:	Lemon Scented Eucalyptus Oil
1.5 AUSTRALIAN AICS Name:	Oils, eucalyptus
1.6 USA INCI Name:	Eucalyptus Citriodora Oil
1.7 EU [Cosing] INCI Name:	Eucalyptus Citriodora Leaf/Twig Oil
1.8 EU [Cosing] Perfuming Name:	Not allocated
1.9 UN Proper Shipping Name:	Environmentally hazardous substance, liquid, n.o.s.
1.10 UN Technical Shipping Name:	[Eucalyptus Citriodora Oil]
1.11 UN Number:	3082
1.12 AUSTRALIAN Schedule Name:	Eucalyptus Oil
1.13 Recommended Product Use:	Cosmetic and aromatherapy ingredient.

Function: Fragrance Ingredient; Skin Conditioning Agent – Miscellaneous.
Categories: Fragrance preparations, miscellaneous; Skin care preparations, miscellaneous.

1.14 Company:	NEW DIRECTIONS AUSTRALIA PTY LTD A.C.N. 052 973 743
1.15 Address:	47 Carrington Road, Marrickville, NSW 2204, AUSTRALIA
1.16 Telephone Number:	+61 2 8577 5999
1.17 Fax Number:	+61 2 8577 5977
1.18 Email:	nda@newdirections.com.au
1.19 Web Site:	www.newdirections.com.au
1.20 Emergency Contact:	Poisons Information Centre Sydney [T] 131126

Let us say you get feedback from a 100 people or more that your natural perfume has helped them with a certain health issue or people love the aroma.

A. Another 100 or more love the fragrance and it becomes very popular.

Then you may want to employ a chemist to do a stability test. That can cost from $1,200 to $5,000 dollars, or more. They only test it for a short period of time.

In both A and B situations you can do a stability test yourself. Document it well.

Natural Compounds are more stable than perfume compounds that you add to creams and alcohol but I still like to test them.

Standard stability test for all fragranced products, not just Fine Fragrances. Take a sample of your fragranced product, and divide into three identical containers.

By Robyn Ji Smith   page. 142

Keep one in the fridge,
One in the dark;
One at a temperature of about 40 deg Celsius;
One at room temperature in the light (maybe on a window sill).

Leave for three months. Three months at 40 deg. C (104degs Fahrenheit) is equivalent to 1 year at room temperature.
Use the sample stored in the fridge as your standard and compare the other two samples for

1. Odour Strength,
2. Odour change,
3. Appearance (e.g. Colour change).

If you want to give marks out of 5, where 1 is "no change" and 5 is totally different. 1,2 and possibly 3, will be acceptable.

If you wish you can use 4 samples keep the 4th at room temperature for 1 year.

I like to keep my samples in a clear glass bottle or jar for easier sight assessment. I then keep them in a brown paper bag to avoid light destroying the essential oil odour molecules.

Add a white swing tag or label to each bottle with your test number and date and add all the info about the tests to a test dairy.

Each time you do a smell test add a date to the tag or label and add notes to the diary.

Perfume Maker Tool Kit

Setup a small **Alchemy** workspace so you always feel enchanted when you work, preferably facing a garden.

Proof Of Natural

If it is a clear glass bottle it is either a synthetic or an alcohol-based liquid, because natural liquids such as essential oil will lose their benefits when exposed to light.
You can also put one drop onto a white piece of paper. When it dries it will leave no mark. But waxes cannot be tested this way so you need suppliers you trust.

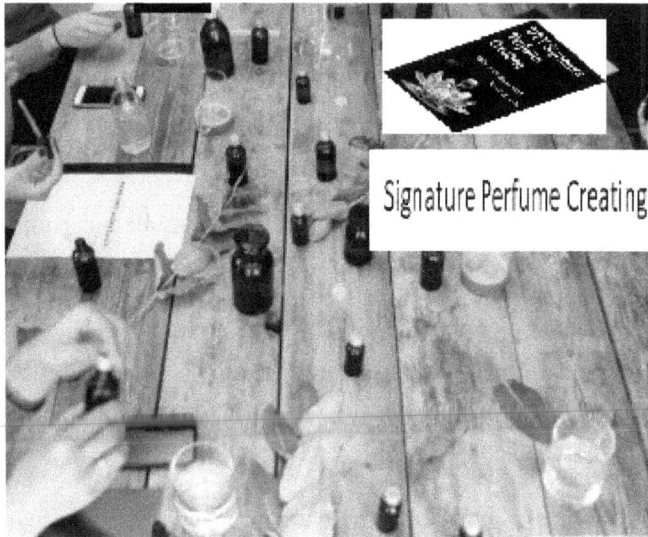

Signature Perfume Creating

A timber book case is a great asset to assist as you can store your bottles, your books, measuring beacons eyedroppers, perfume Samples, Essential oils, test strips, oils and so on.
 A vase of flowers, a desk and your laptop. A timber work table as in this photo is not a sterilized surface. If you work on a timber table or bench top place paper towels or cloth on the work space.

DIY Signature Perfume Creating

Basic Kit List

A basic kit will be as large or as small as you need it to be.

1) 300ml carrier agent (olive oil, grapeseed oil or jojoba oil)
2) 100 ml Fractionated coconut oil
3) 200ml Perfumers alcohol (optional)
4) 1 Perfumer's funnel
5) 20 fragrance tester strips
6) 1 Graduated cylinder
7) 5 x 30ml vials for storing formulas in progress
8) 5 x 10 ml roll-on bottles for oil perfume or
9) 5 off atomizers for alcohol based perfume
10) 5 x 50ml or 100ml Blue, brown or red bottles
11) 8 off 30ml glass bottles with eyedropper or dripper
12) 8 off 10 ml glass bottles with dropper or eyedropper
13) 20 perfume test strips
14) 1 pack Cottonwool pads
15) 1 Roll of paper towel
16) 2 Pair rubber gloves
17) 10 or more pipettes
18) 1 bag Timber stirrers or paddle pop sticks
19) Small glass bowl and saucer
20) A lovely vase
21) Fresh flowers (every time you are working have flowers on your desk.)
22) Apron
23) Safety Glasses from Bunnings
24) Scales
25) Glass stirring rod
26) Peddle bin
27) Pen
28) Pencil
29) Rubber/eraser
30) Tags (white) for bottles. Thick about the size for each bottle size.
31) *Later you will design your signature labels see Marketing.*
32) 8 Essential Oils Or More. *Assorted in top middle and base notes. at least 3 of these should be middle notes, at*

least 3 base notes and the rest should be those enchanting top notes.

33) **Shea Butter -** Refined Certified **or Coconut oil**

34) **One perfume makers diary** for keeping track of your concoctions Just an exercise book is fine. Just but a lined book.

35) **A-Z address** book as well. Once your fragrance has a name add the formula to the address book.

Essential Oils Starter Kit Suggestion

This is a suggestion for your starter kit. However, if you want perfumes for people that have epilepsy, a heart condition or are pregnant you need to understand contra-indications first before buying your kit. Unless you can afford lots of essential oils then you need to choose oils that suit all health conditions. That is covered in the book Called "Foolproof Aromatherapy" By Robyna Smith-Keys.

- Basil *Top to Middle*
- Bergamot *Top*
- Cedarwood (blood) *Base*
- Cinnamon *Base*
- Chamomile *Middle*
- Eucalyptus *Top*
- Frankincense *Base*
- Geranium or Rose Geranium *Middle*
- Ginger Root *Middle*
- Lavender *Top*
- Orange *Top*
- Neroli Blend Top
- Patchouli *Base*
- Petitgrain *Top*
- Vetiver *Base*
- Ylang Ylang Middle to Base

You will organize these in a box of notes. Top Middle and Base notes. Get three children size shoe boxes and organize your oils in boxes labelled Top - Middle - Base

Because Bergamot, Orange and Neroli all come from the orange tree maybe as a start you just can buy one of these oil. They will produce a similar aroma but Bergamot is the most used oil in a fruity fresh designed perfume.

It is entirely up to you what size you buy. However, if you buy - lets say 100ml it is best to decant into several smaller bottles because every time you take the lid off the oil it loses aroma qualities and gains oxygen that will sour the oil... Yet a larger bottle is more economical. Dripolators do help prevent this to some degree.

Three oils that I love to add are

- Rose Geranium
- Rose
- Jasmin

Suppliers

Note: these are not suppliers I am recommending but giving you a mere outline of who is out there to supply you with your needs so you have a base point for your purchases.

Alcohol
https://www.sydneysolvents.com.au/Ethanol-95PGF4-Perfume-Grade-5-Litre

Essential oils and Info
https://www.oilsandplants.com/oils.htm

http://au.springfields.net.au/

Bottles, Essential oils, Talc, Butters

Be Marvelously Alive.   **147** | P a g e

Why Natural Is Best

www.newdirections.com.au

Skin Butters
https://www.awo.com.au/shea-butter-refined-certified-organic-aco-12456/

https://www.creatingperfume.com/PerfumeAlcoholandOils.aspx

Fancy Bottles
http://www.sheleeglass.com/product/
Contact: Elsa Phone: +86 15711809159
E-mail: **xuelee8884@gmail.com**

If buying from Ebay be careful what you are buying I bought blue bottle once and they were painted on the inside. You need bottles that are infused with colour not painted ones.

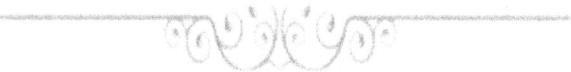

Marketing

Afterpay Available.
Note to students afterpay is an option you should look at when offering products for sale.
https://www.afterpay.com/en-AU/index

For an instant payment I like payments from their mobile phone to mine. You give them your phone number and they get on their phone banking app and send you the money. They then send you the code their bank sent them and they send that to you as a message.
You then open your banking app and put the money into your bank account. It is time consuming but there are no fees to pay.

Also, PayPal is a good provider.

By Robyn Ji Smith   page. 148

https://www.paypal.com/au/home

Payment transfers will depend on what country you reside in. Note Australia was the country chosen to write the international standards for the Beauty Trade. I was an adviser on that panel. Therefore, if you are sticking to natural perfumes you are in safe hands with the information I have provided in this book.

Ready to Launch Your Creation To The World

start with advise here.

The Australian Society of Cosmetic Chemists

https://ascc.com.au/department-of-health-animal-testing-update/

Your Personal Media.

Facebook, Instagram and live chats are good sources

to introduce your perfumes to the public. First be well read on the types of claims you legally can make in your country about your "Natural Perfume". *Remember once you add absolutes or alcohol to your Aroma Base it can no longer be identified as Natural.* Be careful about how you advertise your Perfumes and I am always here to help.

Email beautyschoolbooks@gmail.com

Displays And Storage Boxes.

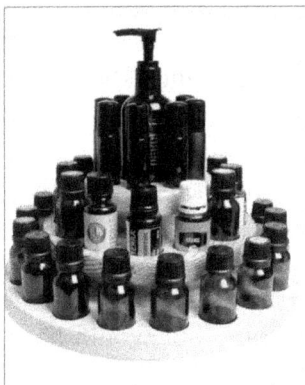

If you consider most of you will start from home and then maybe venture to a market stall, you need to think well in advance about a timber display stand. Therefore, the shelves need to be easily transported.

Timber being such a beautiful natural material would be my first choice. With this in mind consider the sizes of the bottles if you are going to make signature perfumes for individuals on the day. What size your bottles are will be the bases for having a display manufactured.

When working from home you need to be organized.

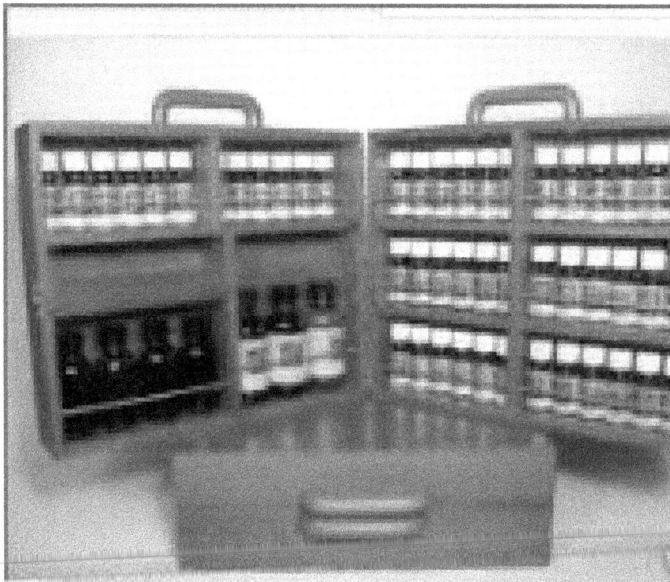

Base oils and bottles will need to have a bigger shelf than your essential oil bottles. Also, because you do not want to worry about the oils being destroyed by light and weather conditions the essential oils should be in dark glass with a pretty label with a dripolator not an eyedropper.

Do not have too many on display as essential oils do not like heat. This wooden display is great for home but would have too many oils on display at a market stall.

However, you could display this many oil bottles with labels but have the bottles empty and the full bottles in an esky.

Do not fill the esky with ice. You could add a cold pack though if it is a hot day. I would not attend markets on heatwave days.

This is where you would do market stalls in winter and only online sales or conduct perfume parties in the summer.

When I did markets, I had a camp fridge in my car. But this also means you need a solar panel and a regulator.

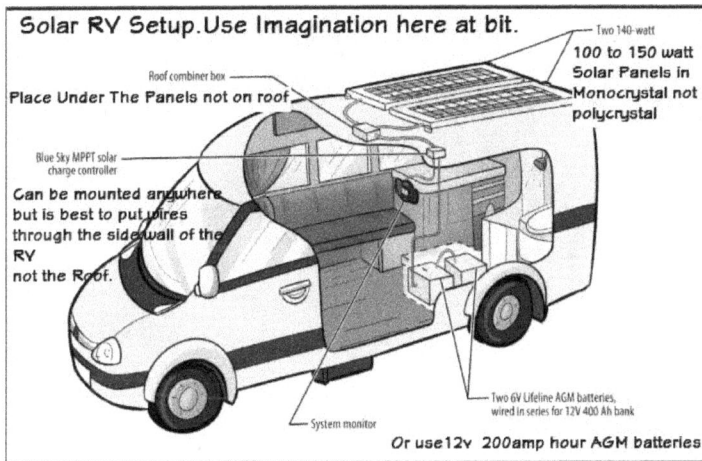

Solar RV Setup. Use Imagination here at bit.

Two 140-watt
100 to 150 watt Solar Panels in Monocrystal not polycrystal

Roof combiner box
Place Under The Panels not on roof

Blue Sky MPPT solar charge controller
Can be mounted anywhere but is best to put wires through the sidewall of the RV not the Roof.

Two 6V Lifeline AGM batteries, wired in series for 12V 400 Ah bank
System monitor

Or use 12v 200amp hour AGM batteries

https://www.facebook.com/photo.php?fbid=10156546038479859&set=g.184346675695363&type=1&theater&ifg=1

Safe Way To Wear Perfume

Offer alternate ways for people to wear perfume.
Timber necklace is one way. Timber holds the aroma for
hours and is a very safe way for people to wear scents. They
place just a few drops on the timber. The perfume aromas also
last longer on timber.

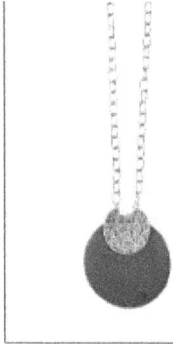

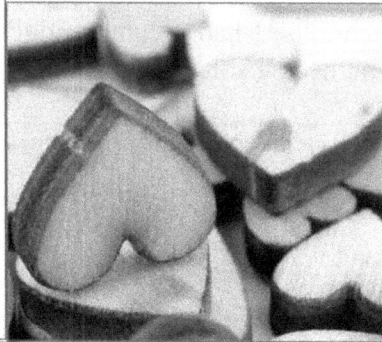

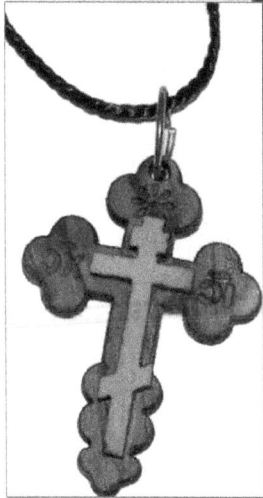

Perfume Lockets

Gold or Silver Lockets in a Filigree Style sometimes come with a velvet lining or do as I do, I put a cotton wool ball inside my gold filigree locket. With perfume on the ball.

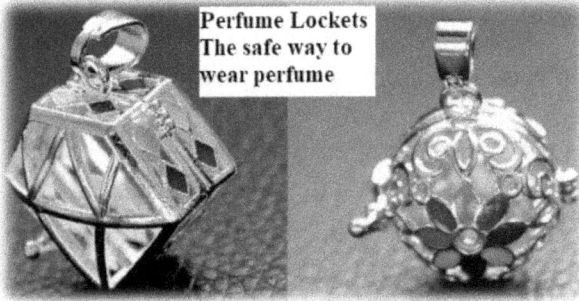

Perfume Lockets
The safe way to
wear perfume

These are a great way to add products to your products for sale list.

Business cards made from white grainy carboard will serve you better than perfume strips for giving people a smell of the fragrance. Tell them it is a handbag aroma card and they keep it. That means sometime later they have all your details and the aroma although slightly milder is still there.

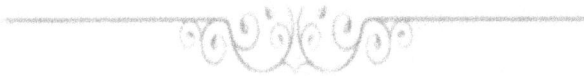

Potpourri And Candles

You may also want to add fragrances to potpourri and candles.

Potpourri
Buy or gather flowers. Dry them or their petal in the sun under a net.
Add a few twigs that you can gather from under trees. Wood holds fragrance 10 times longer than skin or flowers.
Put into a pretty bowl. Spray it with some perfume, and keep its scent going.
You can also spray some Styrofoam packing or dried peanut shells and beach shells with perfume and place them in the bottom of your potpourri bowl.

To add a smaller bowl in the middle filled with bicarbonate of soda it will remove stale odours from the room. Then make a metal cup out of aluminium foil sit it on top of the potpourri with half an onion. The onion will kill bacteria in your home.

Revitalize Dusty Potpourri
Part of keeping your potpourri's scent going strong is keeping it clean. First point of defence against dust is to put a net over the bowl of potpourri.
Here's an easy trick to clean your potpourri: Pour it into a resealable plastic bag, close the top, and use a fork to poke some small holes into the bag. Shake the bag over a garbage can to catch all the dirt and dust that will fall through the holes. Now your potpourri will be as good as new!

Candles
Dig some wax away from near the wick add some essential oils then light the candle. Keep up high away from pets and children. If you have a cat keep an eye on the candle. Perfume compounds can also be sold to candle makers.

Your Labels

If you are going to market your perfumes you will need a professional looking labels. You can make your own or purchase labels.

https://www.ozstickerprinting.com/
https://www.fastprinting.com.au/

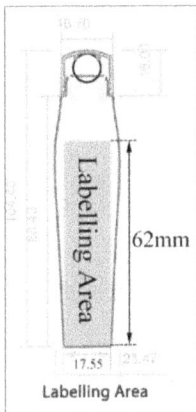

Labelling Area

Note roll-on bottles need a long label due to the shape of the bottle

Possible blurb -

For your perfume making business.

Think clearly about your blurb. Here is a suggestion.

The creation of a fragrance is an excellent example of nature and science working in concert. First you should know I an A trained Hairdresser, Beauty Therapist and have trained hundreds of apprentices and Beauty School students in all elective studies. To add to my credits, I studied Aromatherapy at Nature Care College in Sydney Australia. I am constantly allured by further study of essential oils. I create fragrances from my exquisite collection of pure and natural essences, culled from years of searching for the most beautiful varieties of essential oils. I blend and bottle the fragrances by hand in small batches in my Manly studio a suburb in Sydney Australia. Everything I make is free from synthetics, parabens, glycols, and petrochemicals. However, I do sometimes use wool-fat because it is very close to human skin and its emollient benefits are many. My perfumes and products contain only the purest, most sublime essences from around the world.

I love my small boutique style studio, and work with awe and passion for the alchemy that transforms these rare essences into gorgeous perfumes. They are sold exclusively on my website and are not available in stores. Indulge yourself in Signature Scent: modern natural luxury.

Essential Oil | Boost Immunity The Natural Way
With Over 70 Years' Experience Sourcing & Blending
Natures Most Powerful Essential Oils. Boost Your Immunity
& Relax with Natural Blends Of Premium Quality.

My family made soaps and when I was very young I made them in empty match boxes. There were no essential oils in bottle to purchase in the 1940s so we made natural fragrances at home.

Essential Oils - 100% Cruelty Free. Backed By Science.

Tell people about your journey, about the research you have done or the training you have had.

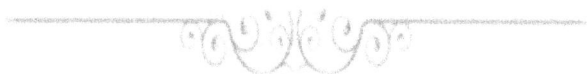

Further reading

Foolproof Aromatherapy by Robyna Smith-Keys
This book cuts to the case it is **not** filled with unessential information and is not loaded with photos. It has condensed information down to the core information required to get the job done. Purchase here
http://www.beautyschoolbooks.com.au/aromatherapy.htm
or Barnes and Noble or Amazon.com.au

https://www.sciencedirect.com/science/article/pii/S0254629910001705

The Olfactory - Smell
https://en.wikipedia.org/wiki/Olfaction#Main_olfactory_system

Musk
https://www.creatingperfume.com/musk.aspx

Other Suggested Reading -
Before Coming To Class- Optional

Robert Tisserand
Robert known as the father of Aromatherapy in Australia now consults to TGA His is passionate about his work and passionate people amazing researchers.
https://tisserandinstitute.org/
https://tisserandinstitute.org/recommended-texts/
https://tisserandinstitute.org/safety/adverse-reaction-database/
https://tisserandinstitute.org/chemistry/

Dr. E. Joy Bowles, PhD, BSc Hons
I myself studied with Joy many decades ago. She is delightful but does talk and ask questions like a scientist. Her books are a must have to understand chemicals in Essential oils.

Why Natural Is Best

https://www.healthline.com

I personally trust the information on this site as they claim to have experts check their documents. You can put the name of the essential oil into their search bar and the information if available will be there.

https://www.awo.com.au/nerolina-essential-oil/

I like how they explain in the description box what oils mix well together. They do not tell you why but if you check your contra-indications of the oils you have further education at you finger tips.

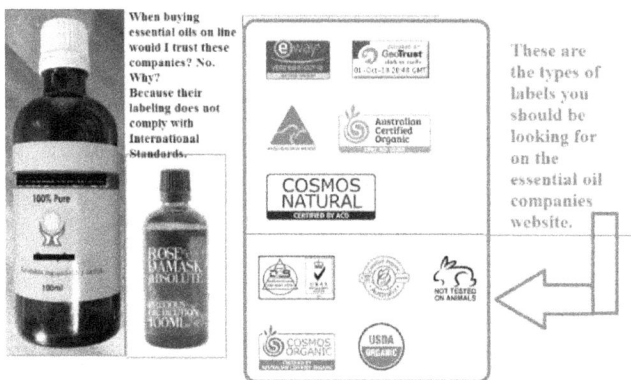

https://www.onlinelabels.com/articles/fda_labeling_requirements.htm

TGA Australia. This is my go to site to keep abreast of what's happening in the industry. This week I had heard on a YouTube video that Rose oil was banned in perfume. As Rose oil has 500 healing properties that set my head in a spin. But as the person telling us this miss information was advertising they would mix safe concentrates for us I was a little sceptical, I was right, pure rose oil is not banned only the synthetic rose was banned.

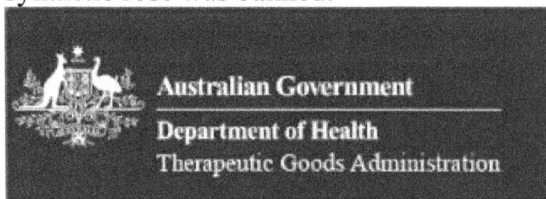

https://search.tga.gov.au/s/search.html?collection=tga-websites-web&query=rose+oil&op=Search

FDA in USA

By Robyn Ji Smith   page. 158

DIY Signature Perfume Creating

https://www.fda.gov/cosmetics/cosmetic-ingredients/fragrances-cosmetics#essential

Labelling Laws Australia and New Zealand
https://www.productsafety.gov.au/standards/cosmetics-ingredients-labelling

Advanced Aromatherapy **(1998) by Dr Kurt Schnaubelt.**

The Practice Of Aromatherapy By Jean Valnet
I love this book it did not give me all I was thirsting for a the time I purchased it (1995) but I could not put it down.

Perfume blog
http://media.allured.com/documents/071112fragrancemythsandfacts.pdf

Essential oil descriptions
https://www.aromaweb.com/essentialoils/default.asp

The Principals and Practice of Perfumery and Cosmetics.
You can borrow this book from Libraries
Here are the libraries that have it in stock in Australia . They will organize it to come to your library for pick up. However, this book is not necessary if you are going to make all natural perfumes.

You can borrow book here Library	
1	State Library of Queensland
	Brisbane, AU-QL 4101 Australia
2	State Library of NSW
	Sydney, AU-NS 2000 Australia
3	Burwood, NSW 2134 Australia
4	State Library of Victoria
	Melbourne, AU-VI 3000 Australia
5	Clarence Regional Library Headquarters

	South Grafton, NSW 2460 Australia
6	Sunshine Coast Libraries
	Nambour, 4560 Australia

Infusing Oils this is a good video

https://www.youtube.com/watch?v=obsj2uL1HNQ

Safety considerations of any wellness tool, including essential oils, is always paramount. This is to achieve the desired responses and avoid any unwanted side effects.

Being mindful of correct dosing and applications can avert potential overdose responses, sensitizations, or interactions.

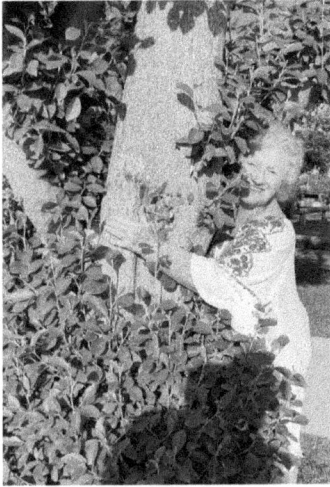

With my love enjoy your new perfume craft.

Hug a tree while you contemplate or meditate

Love Robyn xxx

Keep an eye on my Facebook pages for a new video I will make soon on blending.

I have written several other books 2 that might help you are:-
Alluring Study Of Aromatherapy

Learn Perfume Creating with Natures Gifts

Got It is about dealing with Alcoholics and other difficult people.

DIY Chakra Balancing. Is about connecting to a power greater than yourself.

https://www.facebook.com/groups/FolkloreHealings/

https://www.facebook.com/AromatherapyAndBeautySchoolBooks/

Why Natural Is Best

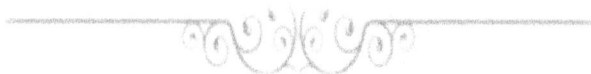

Notes

www.ingramcontent.com/pod-product-compliance
Lightning Source LLC
Chambersburg PA
CBHW080424270326
41929CB00018B/3154